Series Editors:
Steven F. Warren, Ph.D.
Joe Reichle, Ph.D.

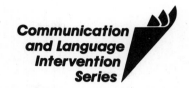
Communication
and Language
Intervention
Series

Volume 4

Specific Language Impairments in Children

Also available in the Communication
and Language Intervention Series:

Volume 1
*Causes and Effects in Communication
and Language Intervention*
edited by Steven F. Warren, Ph.D.
and Joe Reichle, Ph.D.

Volume 2
*Enhancing Children's Communication:
Research Foundations for Intervention*
edited by Ann P. Kaiser, Ph.D.
and David B. Gray, Ph.D.

Volume 3
*Communicative Alternatives
to Challenging Behavior:
Integrating Functional Assessment
and Intervention Strategies*
edited by Joe Reichle, Ph.D.
and David P. Wacker, Ph.D.

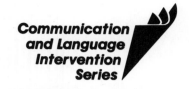

Communication
and Language
Intervention
Series

Volume 4

Specific Language Impairments in Children

Edited by

Ruth V. Watkins, Ph.D.
Assistant Professor
Department of Speech and Hearing Science
University of Illinois, Champaign

and

Mabel L. Rice, Ph.D.
Professor
Department of Speech-Language-Hearing
Director
Child Language Progam
University of Kansas, Lawrence

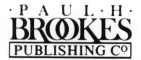

·P·A·U·L·H·
BROOKES
PUBLISHING C<u>O</u>

Baltimore • London • Toronto • Sydney

Paul H. Brookes Publishing Co.
P.O. Box 10624
Baltimore, Maryland 21285-0624

Typeset by The Composing Room of Michigan, Inc., Grand Rapids, Michigan.
Manufactured in the United States of America by
The Maple Press Company, York, Pennsylvania.

This book is printed on recycled paper. ✪

Library of Congress Cataloging-in-Publication Data
Specific language impairments in children / edited by Ruth V. Watkins
and Mabel L. Rice.
    p.   cm — (Communication and language intervention series: 4)
    "Based on papers presented at the 1992 Bruton Conference on
Specific Language Impairments in Children, held at the University of
Texas at Dallas, Callier Center for Communication Disorders"—Pref.
    Includes bibliographical references and index.
    ISBN 1-55766-139-1
    1. Language disorders in children—Congresses. I. Watkins, Ruth
V. II. Rice, Mabel. III. Bruton Conference on Specific Language
Impairments in Children (1992 : Dallas, Tex.) IV. Series.
RJ496.L35S645 1994
618.92′855—dc20   93-39230
                                                  CIP

(British Library Cataloguing-in-Publication data are available from the British
Library.)

Contents

Series Preface

THE PURPOSE OF THE *Communication and Language Intervention Series* is to provide meaningful foundations for the application of sound intervention designs to enhance the development of communication skills across the life span. We are endeavoring to achieve this purpose by providing readers with presentations of state-of-the-art theory, research, and practice.

In selecting topics, editors, and authors, we are not attempting to limit the contents of this series to those viewpoints with which we agree or which we find most promising. We are assisted in our efforts to develop the series by an editorial advisory board consisting of prominent scholars representative of the range of issues and perspectives to be incorporated in the series.

We trust that the careful reader will find much that is provocative and controversial in this and other volumes. This will be necessarily so to the extent that the work reported is truly on the so-called cutting edge, a mythical place where no sacred cows exist. This point is demonstrated time and again throughout this volume as the conventional wisdom is challenged (and occasionally confirmed) by various authors.

Readers of this and other volumes are encouraged to proceed with healthy skepticism. In order to achieve our purpose, we take on some difficult and controversial issues. Errors and misinterpretations are inevitably made. This is normal in the development of any field, and should be welcomed as evidence that the field is moving forward and tackling difficult and weighty issues.

Well-conceived theory and research on development of both children with and children without disabilities is vitally important for researchers, educators, and clinicians committed to the development of optimal approaches to communication and language intervention. For this reason, each volume in this series includes chapters pertaining to both development and intervention.

The content of each volume reflects our view of the symbiotic relationship between intervention and research: Demonstrations of what may work in intervention should lead to analyses of promising discoveries and insights from developmental work that may in turn fuel further refinement and development by intervention researchers.

An inherent goal of this series is to enhance the long-term development of the field by systematically furthering the dissemination of theoretically and empirically based scholarship and research. We promise the reader an opportunity to participate in the development of this field through the debates and discussions that occur throughout the pages of the *Communication and Language Intervention Series*.

Editorial Advisory Board

Volume Preface

THIS VOLUME IS BASED on papers presented at the 1992 Bruton Conference on Specific Language Impairments in Children, held at the University of Texas at Dallas, Callier Center for Communication Disorders. The purpose of this conference was to gather individuals engaged in the study of specific language impairments (SLI) in children for discussion of innovative approaches to research and intervention with this population. Thus, the conference provided an opportunity to highlight the current empirical and conceptual work of scholars in the field of SLI, while integrating the concerns of clinicians working with this population. Conference presenters included: Bruce Tomblin, Martha Crago, Judith Johnston, Mabel Rice, Ruth Watkins, Laurence Leonard, Hugh Catts, Bonnie Brinton, Martin Fujiki, Marc Fey, Alan Kamhi, and Sandy Friel-Patti. Although not all presenters have participated in this volume, the nature and direction of the book have been influenced by the formal and informal exchanges of ideas and information that occurred during the conference. Thus, the contributions of all speakers, as well as conference registrants, are gratefully acknowledged.

Within the volume, three major areas in the current study of SLI are represented. The first is a strong emphasis on the study of genetic contributions to language impairments. Chapters by Tomblin and Buckwalter and Crago and Gopnik (Chapters 2 and 3, respectively) present two different approaches to the study of genetics and SLI. The second major area of study included in the volume is recent advances in characterizing the linguistic profiles of children with SLI. In this area, chapters by Watkins, Rice, and Leonard (Chapters 4, 5, and 6, respectively) highlight varied approaches to documenting the linguistic manifestations of SLI and alternative frameworks through which these linguistic profiles can be organized, interpreted, and evaluated. The third major area of investigation included in the volume addresses the challenges facing children with SLI in related domains. Johnston (Chapter 7) focuses on cognitive abilities in children with SLI, and Fey, Long, and Cleave (Chapter 10) examine links between cognitive skills, grammatical abilities, and intervention effectiveness with the SLI population. In turn, Fujiki and Brinton (Chapter 8) examine the relation between language and social competence in children with SLI, while Catts, Hu, Larrivee, and Swank (Chapter 9) address ties between early speech and language impairments and subsequent reading disorders.

Although many important aspects of the study of SLI are represented in this volume, a number of relevant avenues of investigation are also notably absent. There is a rapidly growing body of literature from diverse fields addressing SLI; it was not possible to include all pertinent areas of inquiry within this book. Chapter 1 (Watkins) provides an introduction to the study of SLI, highlights material included as well as excluded from this text, and outlines the general framework of the book. As one of a very small set of texts devoted to the field of SLI, this volume represents significant progress in our knowledge, understanding, and awareness of the disorder. This volume seeks to contribute to the interpretation of innovative research findings, as well as to the quality and direction of future empirical investigations and clinical practice in the area of SLI.

Contributors

The Editors

Ruth V. Watkins, Ph.D., Assistant Professor, Department of Speech and Hearing Science, University of Illinois, 901 South Sixth Street, Champaign, IL 61820. Dr. Watkins's research has focused on characterizing the linguistic deficits of children with SLI, and on approaches to intervention with young children with language impairments. Her previous faculty appointment was in the School of Human Development, University of Texas at Dallas.

Mabel L. Rice, Ph.D., Professor, Department of Speech-Language-Hearing, University of Kansas, 1082 Dole Hall, Lawrence, KS 66045. Dr. Rice is also Director of the Child Language Program and the Kansas Early Childhood Research Institute at the University of Kansas. Her current research addresses many aspects of SLI, including morphological and syntactic deficits, lexical learning, social and academic consequences, and approaches to preschool language intervention.

The Chapter Authors

Bonnie Brinton, Ph.D., Associate Professor, Speech-Language Pathology Area, Educational Psychology Department, Brigham Young University, P.O. Box 28713, Provo, UT 84602. Dr. Brinton's research has examined a wide range of topics related to conversational language impairment in children with language disorders and adults with mental retardation.

Paula R. Buckwalter, M.S., Research Assistant, Department of Speech-Language Pathology, University of Iowa, Iowa City, IA 52242. Mrs. Buckwalter's research focuses on the identification and causes of speech-language impairment. She is currently conducting a twin study of SLI.

Hugh W. Catts, Ph.D., Associate Professor, Department of Speech-Language-Hearing, University of Kansas, 3031 Dole Hall, Lawrence, KS 66045. Dr. Catts's research interests include the early identification and remediation of language-based reading disabilities. He has published a book on this topic, with colleague Dr. Alan Kamhi.

Patricia L. Cleave, M.Cl.Sc., Research Assistant, Department of Speech-Language-Hearing, University of Kansas, 3031 Dole Hall, Lawrence, KS 66045. Ms. Cleave is currently a doctoral student at the University of Kansas, with research interests in the areas of morphological and lexical acquisition in children with specific language impairment. Ms. Cleave's work also addresses treatment efficacy in the area of preschool language intervention.

Martha B. Crago, Ph.D., Assistant Professor, School of Human Communication Disorders, McGill University, 1266 Pine Avenue West, Montreal, Quebec H3G 1A8, Canada. Dr. Crago is involved in a spectrum of research that addresses both the innate and the socially constructed properties of language. She is presently engaged in cross-linguistic research on family aggregations with specific language impairment and in a series of language socialization studies that take place in the homes and schools of Inuit, Cree, Mohawk, and Algonquin communities.

Marc E. Fey, Ph.D., Associate Professor, Hearing and Speech Department, University of Kansas Medical Center, 3901 Rainbow Boulevard, Kansas City, KS 66160. Dr. Fey's research and clinical interests focus primarily on preschool- and early school-age children with language and/or phonological impairments. Dr. Fey's studies have addressed a wide range of topics in the area of language impairments in children, with particular emphasis on the experimental evaluation of treatment efficacy.

Martin Fujiki, Ph.D., Associate Professor, Speech-Language Pathology Area, Educational Psychology Department, Brigham Young University, P.O. Box 28673, Provo, UT 84602. Dr. Fujiki's research activities address conversational language difficulties in children with language impairment and adults with mental retardation.

Myrna Gopnik, Ph.D., Professor, Department of Linguistics, McGill University, 1001 Sherbrooke Street West, Montreal, Quebec H3A IG5, Canada. Dr. Gopnik's work focuses on characterizing the linguistic properties of genetically impaired language development within a principled linguistic framework. She is also engaged in a long-term research project to investigate a wide range of linguistic properties across several languages.

Chieh-Fang Hu, Ph.D., Child Language Program, University of Kansas, 1082 Dole Hall, Lawrence, KS 66045. Dr. Hu recently completed her doctoral degree at the University of Kansas. Her research addresses phonological processing in beginning readers of Chinese.

Judith R. Johnston, Ph.D., Professor and Director, School of Audiology and Speech Sciences, University of British Colombia, 5804 Fairview Avenue, Vancouver, British Colombia V6T 1Z3, Canada. Dr. Johnston's research is focused on the evolving relationships between cognition and language in young children. As one approach to this problem, she has investigated cognitive abilities in children whose language and cognitive development are dissociated, such as children with specific language impairment. Dr. Johnston also teaches courses in developmental language intervention and directs a professional education program. In these endeavors, she attempts to translate the knowledge and perspectives of disciplines such as psycholinguistics into principles for clinical practice.

Linda Larrivee, M.S., Research Assistant, Department of Speech-Language-Hearing, University of Kansas, 2101 Haworth Hall, Lawrence, KS 66045. Ms. Larrivee is a doctoral student at the University of Kansas, with extensive clinical experience in promoting the language skills of children with language-learning disabilities. Her research interests include language impairments and reading disabilities in school-age children.

Laurence B. Leonard, Ph.D., Distinguished Professor, Department of Audiology and Speech Sciences, Purdue University, Heavilon Hall, West Lafayette, IN 47907.

Dr. Leonard's research is concerned with the syntactic, morphological, semantic, and phonological abilities of children with language disorders. His most recent work has focused on cross-linguistic comparisons of children with specific language impairment.

Steven H. Long, Ph.D., Postdoctoral Trainee, Department of Speech and Hearing Sciences, University of Washington, Eagleson Hall, JG-15, Seattle, WA 98195. Dr. Long's studies have examined both typical and impaired lexical and grammatical development in preschoolers. Dr. Long has also explored methods for transcribing and analyzing spontaneous language sample data, including development of a set of computerized modules to assist in the analysis of speech and language transcripts.

Linda Swank, Ph.D., Assistant Professor, Human Services and Communication Disorders Program, University of Virginia, P.O. Box 9022, Charlottesville, VA 22906. Dr. Swank's research interests include a number of topics related to language-based reading disorders, including phonological impairments, phonological awareness and coding, morphophonemic development, word retrieval, and vocabulary acquisition. Dr. Swank also serves as the Director of the University of Virginia Language-Based Reading Disorders Clinic.

J. Bruce Tomblin, Ph.D., Professor, Department of Speech-Language Pathology and Audiology, University of Iowa, Iowa City, IA 52242. Dr. Tomblin's research is concerned with identifying and understanding those factors that predispose and cause SLI. In particular, he is attempting to understand why SLI runs in families and the manner in which genes contribute to this familiality.

Acknowledgments

THIS VOLUME WAS PREPARED as a result of the 1992 Bruton Conference on Specific Language Impairments in Children, held at the University of Texas at Dallas, Callier Center for Communication Disorders. The conference was underwritten by the David Bruton, Jr., Endowment Fund. We are very grateful to the David Bruton family for supporting the conference, and enabling the scientific and clinical insights that developed from it. Over the past 10 years, the Bruton Endowment has promoted the exchange of innovative research and clinical knowledge at the University of Texas at Dallas. We are pleased to acknowledge the contribution of the Bruton Endowment to the conference and this volume, recognizing that the exchange of knowledge that occurred will lead to improved clinical service delivery for young children with language impairments and will enhance research efforts in the area.

We also extend appreciation to Kathy Hogan and Claudia Davis for their assistance in conference organization. Their planning and management of conference details made an invaluable contribution to the success of the event.

Specific Language Impairments
in Children

1

Specific Language
Impairments in Children

An Introduction

Ruth V. Watkins

T HE BOUNDARIES OF contemporary studies of specific language impairment (SLI) are perhaps most clearly defined by the 1960 Institute on Childhood Aphasia, which offered an exclusionary definition of the disorder that continues to be useful and pertinent (Johnston, 1988). In brief, SLI was defined as delayed acquisition of language skills, occurring in conjunction with normal functioning in intellectual, social-emotional, and auditory domains.

Parallel with the study of language acquisition in children without disabilities, research addressing the nature, character, and cause of SLI has expanded rapidly over the years since the meeting of the Institute on Childhood Aphasia. During this period, study of SLI has evolved into a rich and informative area of scientific inquiry. Furthermore, examination of SLI is timely, insofar as research findings provide insights for current models of language acquisition and impairment and simultaneously contribute to our knowledge of valid and effective approaches to language facilitation.

This volume, focusing entirely on SLI, represents both the timeliness and potential contribution of study in this domain. Throughout the volume, however, two related issues reveal that focused, scientific examination of SLI is both relatively young and rather diffuse. First, although many aspects of SLI have been studied and multiple explanations have been offered for various patterns of linguistic, cognitive, and social performance within this population, myriad questions remain unresolved. For example, we have yet to establish a widely accepted profile of linguistic behavior consistently associated with the disorder. Moreover, multiple causal explanations for SLI have been advanced; although many such explanations enjoy some support in the presently available data, most suffer also from certain inconsistencies or, minimally, remain to be delineated fully (see Bishop, 1992; Johnston, 1988; Leonard, 1987; Rice, 1991, for more complete reviews).

Second, investigators have approached the study of SLI from a variety of disciplines, armed with a diverse array of theoretical models. SLI has been investigated by developmental and experimental psychologists, linguists, psycholinguists, speech-language pathologists, and special educators, among others. One consequence of this diversity is the application of competing theoretical models to account for data from children with SLI; various models have been employed, and, on occasion, stretched to fit the study of SLI in a manner beyond their original scope and intention. For example, recent explanations of the language profiles evident in children with SLI have drawn upon competing linguistic models, such as universal grammar (Chomsky, 1981; cf. Clahsen, 1989, 1991) and learnability theory (Pinker, 1984, 1989a, 1989b; cf. Leonard, 1989). In some cases, divergent models have been applied within a single account of the difficulties of children with SLI (Gopnik & Crago, 1991). Clearly, theoretical models inform the study of SLI, and, in turn, the profile of SLI is pertinent to the development of accurate and appropriate accounts of language acquisition. However, the diversity of models employed in the study of SLI lends additional complexity to interpreting current research in the area.

As a means to recognizing the diversity of relevant models and issues in the study of SLI, this chapter serves as a general introduction to the volume. The chapter begins with a discussion of the fundamental issues in the area of SLI, including approaches to defining the disorder and recent perspectives on its causes and consequences. Then, major areas of current investigation within the SLI field are outlined, highlighting the aims and contributions of the work presented in this text.

FUNDAMENTAL ISSUES IN THE STUDY OF SLI

Definition and Characteristics

As mentioned above, SLI generally has not been defined by what it *is*, but rather, but what it *is not*. Stark and Tallal (1981) provided the accepted standard in terms of SLI definition, particularly for the purposes of empirical research. Stark and Tallal labeled as SLI those children who displayed standardized language test scores at least 12 months below chronological or mental age. They then excluded children who demonstrated any of the following: 1) hearing thresholds above 25 dB HL, 2) parent or teacher report of significant emotional or behavior problems, 3) performance IQ = −1.00 standard deviation or below, 4) evidence of frank neurological deficits, and 5) severe articulation/phonological deficits. Most subsequent studies have employed some variation of these criteria in investigations of the linguistic, social, and cognitive abilities of children with SLI.

In recent years, updates and alternatives to the basic definitional criteria developed by Stark and Tallal (1981) have been offered (cf. Lahey, 1990).

One such alternative is subtyping. It is generally accepted by clinicians and researchers alike that considerable diversity is present across children identified with SLI; much heterogeneity exists in the behavioral profiles and manifestations associated with SLI. For example, children with SLI may vary in the extent of linguistic impairment they exhibit, in the range of linguistic subsystems involved (i.e., semantics, syntax, pragmatics, phonology), and in the modality affected (i.e., expressive vs. receptive deficits). There have been several attempts to describe this diversity, in the form of identifying discrete subtypes or profiles of language impairment (e.g., Aram & Nation, 1975; Rapin & Allen, 1983; Wilson & Risucci, 1986). Aram and Nation identified six discrepant patterns of language deficit (e.g., generalized expressive deficiency, uniform deficiency for all language tasks), whereas Rapin and Allen delineated seven different subtypes (e.g., phonological-syntactic syndrome). It should be noted that the particular patterns of language impairment identified differed across studies.

Despite recognition of heterogeneity of children with SLI, none of the subtyping approaches has gained general acceptance or widespread use; accurate and complete characterization of the diversity of children with SLI via subtyping remains illusive. To date, few studies of children with SLI have used subtypes to identify or describe subjects. This is not to suggest that additional speculation of children who demonstrate varied patterns of language problems is not important (Aram, Morris, & Hall, 1993). The key issue is identifying the most useful and informative way to proceed. One suggestion offered by Aram et al. is the complete specification of subjects with SLI in research reports. This information may serve to promote knowledge of various patterns of language problems.

An additional historical issue in identification and description of children with SLI is that of delay versus deviance. In brief, the basic controversy is whether children with SLI exhibit protracted acquisition of language while following typical developmental patterns, or if the language learning of children with SLI is better characterized by different developmental sequences and processes (Curtiss, Katz, & Tallal, 1992). Many investigations of the linguistic skills of children with SLI have been framed as contributing to the delay–deviance debate (Curtiss et al., 1992; Johnston & Kamhi, 1984; Lahey, Liebergott, Chesnick, Menyuk, & Adams, 1992; Leonard, 1972, 1979); most have used a three-group research design wherein youngsters with SLI are compared with two groups of typically developing peers, one equated with the SLI group on the basis of age, the other on general language ability (usually via mean length of utterance). The logic here is that deviant language acquisition should be revealed in cases where children with SLI perform more poorly than language-equivalent peers. In contrast, linguistic performance that equals language-mates suggests delayed development.

Results of these investigations have been mixed. Perhaps the strongest support for deviant patterns of acquisition comes from evidence in the domains of syntax and morphology. For example, one of the most consistently documented characteristics of SLI is difficulty in the acquisition of grammatical morphology (Clahsen, 1989, 1991; Crago & Gopnik, 1994; Gopnik, 1990a, 1990b; Gopnik & Crago, 1991; Khan & James, 1983; Leonard, Bortolini, Caselli, McGregor, & Sabbadini, 1992; Leonard, Sabbadini, Volterra, & Leonard, 1988; Rice & Oetting, 1993; Steckol & Leonard, 1979). Furthermore, a number of other areas of grammar have been shown to be less advanced in children with SLI than in their language-equivalent counterparts (e.g., syntactic complexity, Chiat & Hirson, 1987; Johnston & Kamhi, 1984; verb particles, Watkins & Rice, 1991; aspects of derivational morphology, Watkins, Buhr, & Davis, 1993). However, some discrepancy exists between these relatively focused findings and more general investigations. For example, Curtiss et al. (1992) examined the performance of children with SLI in both receptive and expressive domains on a diverse set of syntactic skills (subtests of the *CYCLE* were used, Curtiss & Yamada, 1988). Overall, they found a pattern of general similarity between children with SLI and their language-equivalent peers in terms of rate and sequence of acquisition.

Results from other domains of language are also equivocal. In terms of the lexicon, for example, some studies have demonstrated that children with SLI show acquisition patterns that parallel those of their typically developing counterparts, but occur more slowly (cf. Camarata & Schwartz, 1985; Leonard, 1988). However, recent investigations indicate that acquisition of a main verb lexicon may be particularly vulnerable in children with SLI (Fletcher, 1993; Fletcher & Peters, 1984; Rice & Bode, 1993; Watkins, Rice, & Moltz, 1993).

Thus, the question of whether the linguistic skills of children with SLI are characterized best as delayed or deviant remains unresolved. Findings may differ, given the domain of study, and the nature of the investigation in question. It seems likely that the ultimate solution to this puzzle will be complex and not as straightforward as the original assumptions of the delayed or deviant framing. The product of this inquiry, however, is a rich and informative, if diverse, knowledge base. These investigations have helped delineate the nature and character of SLI and have contributed to our understanding of the disorder well beyond the basic delay–deviance question.

Consequences

Clinicians have long reported that many children identified and served as SLI in the preschool years reemerge as language-impaired and/or language-learning disabled in the school years (Wallach & Miller, 1988). A more specific issue is the finding that aspects of the linguistic profile of SLI may continue into adulthood. Recent evidence demonstrates that early language impairments can persist, with certain characteristics of SLI, such as difficulty in productively controlling use of grammatical morphemes, constituting particular and continued difficulty (Gopnik & Crago, 1991; Tomblin, Freese, & Records, 1990, 1992). Thus, the implications of SLI can be far-reaching.

A growing body of work also suggests that what seems to begin as an impairment specific to language, ultimately has the potential to influence a wide range of developmental domains. One major area of investigation has explored the link between early language impairments and later reading and academic difficulties. In brief, this work demonstrates that children with SLI are vulnerable to difficulties in successfully making the transition from oral to written language (Catts, 1993; Kamhi & Catts, 1986, 1989). As a group, children with SLI have a significant likelihood of experiencing reading difficulties and associated academic failure (Catts, 1993; Wallach & Butler, 1984; Wallach & Miller, 1988).

A second line of inquiry has examined the social interactive skills of children with SLI (Brinton & Fujiki, 1989). Rice and her colleagues have completed a series of studies examining the social interactions of children with SLI and their peers without disabilities in a preschool classroom (Gertner, 1993; Hadley & Rice, 1991; Rice, 1993; Rice, Sell, & Hadley, 1991). These investigations revealed that children with SLI are more likely to be ignored in conversation by their counterparts without disabilities, and they are less likely to be identified as preferred playmates (Gertner, 1993; Hadley & Rice, 1991). Furthermore, Rice, Hadley, and Alexander (1993) investigated the extent to which kindergarten teachers' expectations and perceptions were influenced by children's expressive language and speech skills. Findings indicated that children with limitations in language and/or speech ability were perceived as less skilled in a number of academic and social areas relative to their peers without disabilities (e.g., perceived to be less intelligent, less likely to be leaders, less popular, less mature).

In summary, it is clear that SLI can be associated with negative developmental consequences in a number of domains throughout the school years and into adulthood. Recent investigations suggest that difficulties in language learning can persist beyond childhood, and that these difficulties are likely to be linked to reading/academic problems and social bias.

Etiology

In parallel with research focusing on characteristics and consequences of SLI, significant effort has been directed toward identifying the source of the disorder. As is the case for many issues in the field, the study of SLI etiology has sparked much debate, and it has spawned many diverse perspectives. Three major hypotheses were reviewed by Leonard (1987). Two of these, the cognitive/representational hypothesis and the auditory perception theory, suggest that the source of the deficit lies within the child; the third points to flaws in the child's communicative environment as the cause of the disorder. Each of these is briefly discussed.

In the cognitive/representational hypothesis, subtle deficits in mental representation ability, differences not detected by nonverbal intelligence measures, are proposed to be responsible for the language-learning problems of children with SLI (Johnston, 1988, 1991a; Johnston & Smith, 1989; Nelson, Kamhi, & Apel, 1987; Terrell, Schwartz, Prelock, & Messick, 1984). The auditory perception account posits that children with SLI have difficulties in perceiving rapid acoustic events. According to this account, children with SLI are less skilled than their peers in processing auditory information of brief duration relative to surrounding segments (Tallal, 1976; Tallal & Piercy, 1973; Tallal, Stark, Kallman, & Mellits, 1981). Finally, the environmental input view holds that the linguistic deficits of children with SLI can be attributed to a degraded communicative environment; central to this view is the idea that children with SLI do not receive the amount and type of linguistic input necessary for optimal language acquisition (Cramblit & Siegel, 1977; Cross, Nienhuys, & Kirkman, 1985; Lasky & Klopp, 1982).

Evaluating these accounts of SLI etiology, Leonard (1987) reported that each perspective has weaknesses. The account with the least empirical support is the environmental input perspective; essentially no evidence exists to suggest that parental input differences are responsible for children's language-learning deficits (Conti-Ramsden, 1990; Lederberg, 1980; Leonard, 1987). In terms of the mental representation account, Leonard (1987) indicated that because SLI children performed better than language-matched peers on many tasks, the power of this account was limited. Finally, the primary flaw of the auditory perception account was that, although difficulties in processing rapid auditory information have been consistently documented, the account does not present a well-integrated whole that can, with clarity, account for the full range of linguistic problems evident in children with SLI.

The limitations of these accounts of SLI seem to have served as catalysts for recent developments in the field. First, several more specific, localized accounts of SLI have been offered. For example, a number of accounts of deficits of children with SLI in the domain of grammatical morphology have been offered. These include Leonard's (1989) surface account and Gopnik and Crago's (1991) missing features hypothesis (see also Crago & Gopnik, chap. 3, this volume; Leonard, chap. 6, this volume); additional accounts include Clahsen's (1989, 1991) proposal that children with SLI are impaired in their ability to form agreement relations within the grammar, and Rice's (chap. 5, this volume) functional category accounts of the morphological deficits of children with SLI. Each of these accounts hypothesizes either a fundamental impairment in the underlying linguistic mechanisms in children with SLI, or suggests limitations in their language-processing aptitude; however, the particular mechanism or ability invoked differs widely across accounts. The scope of these accounts is significantly more focused than the global perspectives outlined above, and each has the strength of a direct link to documented linguistic deficits of children with SLI. Each also makes specific predictions and permits empirical evaluation of its accuracy and completeness. Ultimately, the complete package of strengths and weaknesses associated with SLI must be accounted for. Given the scope of this task, however, more circumscribed accounts offer a positive approach.

Moreover, questions surrounding etiology have led to a general evaluation of the value and feasibility of identifying the cause of SLI. A recent clinical forum published in *Language, Speech and Hearing Services in the Schools* presented a wide spectrum of views on the issue (cf. Aram, 1991; Dale & Cole, 1991; Johnston, 1991b; Leonard, 1991; Tomblin, 1991). The debate centered on the ideas of Leonard (1991), who suggested that a language impairment represents the low end of the normal continuum of linguistic aptitude, and does not embody a particularly different set of learning skills or mechanisms. The child with SLI simply has received a weak set of the attributes that lead to normal variation in language proficiency. For this reason, Leonard proposed that research seeking the source of SLI may not be fruitful.

Leonard's comments sparked a range of responses from colleagues whose work focuses on children with SLI. Aram (1991) and Tomblin (1991) offered rationales for the importance of continuing to pursue the etiology of SLI. Both authors emphasized the clinical relevance of seeking causality (e.g., parent counseling, treatment decision making), and suggested that determining causality is central to advancing the study of SLI as an area of scientific inquiry. Aram also highlighted the fact that, rather than one causal factor involved in SLI, multiple causal factors may well be implicated; furthermore, Aram suggested that the shortcomings of available etiological theories are tied to the fact that most investigations have proceeded as if a single causal factor could be identified (cf. Aram et al., 1993). In turn, although Johnston (1991b) concurred with Leonard that SLI children may well represent the lowest end of the normal distribution of language acquisition, she concluded that the pursuit of causality is both important and likely to be productive. In Johnston's (1991b) view, the constellation of strengths and weaknesses present in children with SLI provides a unique opportunity to scrutinize the links between verbal and nonverbal abilities.

Thus, the varied perspectives on the value of pursuing the etiology of SLI have diverging implications for the nature and direction of future work. Given Leonard's (1991) orientation, a detailed description and synthesis of the nature of impaired language is imperative, and it promises to be more informative than continuing the search for etiology. In turn, researchers in accord with Aram's (1991) and Tomblin's (1991) views will vigorously pursue research emphasizing causal factors in SLI.

CONTEMPORARY STUDY OF SLI: AN OUTLINE OF THIS VOLUME

The divergence in approach to causal factors in SLI has, in fact, led to varied directions in contemporary research on the disorder. Three key areas of study have been advanced. First, investigators committed to the central importance of etiology have extended the traditional boundaries of causal research in new directions, chiefly to the study of genetic and neurological contributions to SLI. Second, researchers less invested in the potential informativeness of etiologic study have approached the problem from an alternative direction, that is, by providing detailed descriptions of the linguistic manifestations of the disorder, and by framing these descriptions within linguistic models. The aim of this work is not unrelated to the first objective, in that descriptions of the problem may ultimately provide key knowledge of the behavioral profile associated with a genetic difficulty. Advancing a third approach to the study of SLI, scholars have sought a better understanding of the scope of the disorder by examining the skills of children with SLI in related areas, as well as assessing how basic characteristics associated with the disorder relate to language skills and treatment outcomes.

Although this volume does not attempt to present the complete body of available research in these areas, each of the three central avenues of study is represented. This volume provides a forum for integrating current approaches to the investigation and understanding of SLI; our rationale is that the clearest understanding of SLI will be generated from integrating the findings of divergent approaches to the study of the disorder. A general outline of research in each area is presented.

Genetic Characterizations

Recent investigations of causal factors in SLI have focused on the rich and informative area of genetic aspects of the disorder. A variety of research methods have been implemented, including case studies (Gopnik, 1990a), family studies (Crago & Gopnik, chap. 3, this volume; Gopnik & Crago, 1991), and large-scale group investigations (Tallal, Ross, & Curtiss, 1989; Tallal, Townsend, Curtiss, & Wulfeck, 1991; Tomblin, 1989). Two key aspects of this groundbreaking work appear in this volume: Crago and Gopnik's detailed investigation of one extended family with a strong history of SLI (Chapter 3); and Tomblin and Buckwalter's epidemiological studies of familiality and heritability of SLI (Chapter 2). Although Crago and Gopnik and Tomblin and Freese share the goal of identifying a genetic underpinning for SLI, they differ markedly in their approaches to this objective. Crago and Gopnik contrast the linguistic profiles of a single family whose members are identified as affected with SLI or nonaffected, and they attempt to delineate possible modes of transmission of the disorder within this family. In contrast, Tomblin and Buckwalter investigate familiality, linguistic profiles, and possible modes of transmission of SLI across a large number of families.

In addition to the work in this volume, several other aspects of investigation in this area are noteworthy. First, a number of recent advances have occurred in the study of the genetic basis of a range of speech, language, and reading disorders (Lewis, 1990, 1993; Lewis, Ekelman, & Aram, 1989; Ludlow & Cooper, 1983; Neils & Aram, 1986; Parlour, 1990; Pennington, 1989). Furthermore, advances in the study of neurology suggest that genetic contributions to SLI may be realized in neuroanatomical differences (Plante, 1991; Plante, Swisher, Vance, & Rapcsak, 1991). This work is preliminary in nature; nevertheless, available results and enhanced methods of study suggest a promising area for further investigation.

Linguistic Description

As summarized above, research and theory in this area seek to describe the linguistic manifestations of SLI, and fit identified strengths and weaknesses to varied linguistic models. Leonard's (1989) low phonetic substance or surface hypothesis is representative of this work; in the hypothesis, Leonard (1989) suggested that children with SLI have difficulty in perceiving, processing, and building generalized linguistic rules for low phonetic substance aspects of the grammar (i.e., elements of brief duration and limited stress). This account was constructed to describe the patterns of difficulty for acquisition of grammatical morphology in children with SLI, and it has been extended to and evaluated against cross-linguistic patterns of morpheme acquisition in children with the disorder.

Contrasting characterization of the morphological deficits in children with SLI has been offered by Clahsen (1989, 1991), Gopnik and Crago (1991), and Rice (chap. 5, this volume). Although these descriptions draw on diverging linguistic models and theoretical orientations, research in this area shares the goal of fully characterizing the linguistic problems associated with SLI. In this volume, Watkins (Chapter 4) summarizes findings from three investigations of the grammatical challenges facing children with SLI. These challenges are then related to existing accounts of the deficits of children with SLI, and areas of compatibility and incompatibility are identified. Similarly, Rice (chap. 5, this volume) reviews data on the mastery of two grammatical morphemes in children with SLI, contrasts these findings with available accounts of their morphological deficits, and proposes two alternative models designed to illuminate plausible underlying grammars of children with SLI. Finally, Leonard (chap. 6, this volume) discusses the limitations of available approaches to accounting for the morphological deficits of children with SLI and suggests research approaches to ameliorate these difficulties.

Competencies in Related Areas

Recent advances in understanding the abilities and disabilities of children with SLI in a number of areas related to the acquisition of language are also addressed in this volume. Although a wide range of research in associated areas could be presented here, competencies in the areas of cognitive, social, and reading ability are highlighted. Johnston (chap. 7, this volume) provides a summary of her research and that of her colleagues dealing with the non-linguistic cognitive skills of children with SLI. In brief, Johnston's perspective is that language and cognitive abilities are closely tied; language deficits both reflect and direct subtle cognitive weaknesses. The work of Fey, Long, and Cleave (chap. 10, this volume) also addresses issues related to cognitive skills in children with SLI, chiefly links between IQ, grammatical characteristics, responses to intervention. Fey et al. also describe two effective approaches to grammatical intervention with children with SLI.

Fujiki and Brinton (chap. 8, this volume) address the complex interaction of linguistic and social competence in children with SLI and review research that reveals the social risk present for children with SLI. In turn, Catts, Hu, Larrivee, and Swank (chap. 9, this volume) present new findings on the link between early speech and language problems and later reading difficulties; more specifically, Catts et al. delineate the tie between phonologic awareness skills and word recognition and decoding abilities.

SUMMARY

In brief, this book offers innovative research in the field of SLI, and reviews fundamental insights provided by current science in the area. The diversity of topics addressed and the models invoked reflect the state of practice in the study of SLI. We do not intend to examine all pertinent work in the field exhaustively; instead, we synthesize the important empirical findings and theoretical orientations. Although we emphasize that which is revealed in these findings and ideas, perhaps more importantly we shift our attention toward identifying critical questions and directions for future research.

Ultimately, one of the most critical questions raised in this volume is why investigation of SLI is a significant area of scientific inquiry. At least two answers to this question are clear. First, from a theoretical perspective, exploration and knowledge of SLI broadens our understanding of the nature and character of language, the mechanisms of language learning, and the associations between various facets of the human mind. Second, as clinical scientists, we seek to identify those aspects of the linguistic system that are most disrupted and examine why they are, what the long-term implications of a language impairment are, whether and which language competencies can be taught, and which methods of language facilitation may lead to optimal outcomes. With regard to clinical concerns, it should be noted that this volume does not contain a section exclusively devoted to consideration of clinical issues. Instead, each author addresses the clinical implications that stem from his or her empirical findings or theoretical orientation. The assumption is that sound clinical strategies and practices are empirically derived, and that they are best presented and interpreted within that context.

REFERENCES

Aram, D.M. (1991). Comments on specific language impairment as a clinical category. *Language, Speech and Hearing Services in the Schools, 22,* 84–87.

Aram, D.M., Morris, R., & Hall, N.E. (1993). Clinical and research congruence in identifying children with specific language impairment. *Journal of Speech and Hearing Research, 36,* 580–591.

Aram, D.M., & Nation, J.E. (1975). Patterns of language behavior in children with developmental language disorders. *Journal of Speech and Hearing Disorders, 18,* 229–241.

Bishop, D.V.M. (1992). The underlying nature of specific language impairment. *Journal of Child Psychology & Psychiatry & Allied Disciplines, 33*(1), 3–66.

Brinton, B., & Fujiki, M. (1989). *Conversational management with language-impaired children.* Rockville, MD: Aspen.

Camarata, S., & Schwartz, R. (1985). Production of object words and action words: Evidence for a relationship between phonology and semantics. *Journal of Speech and Hearing Research, 28,* 323–330.

Catts, H.W. (1993). The relationship between speech-language impairments and reading disabilities. *Journal of Speech and Hearing Research, 36,* 948–958.

Chiat, S., & Hirson, A. (1987). From conceptual intention to utterance: A study of impaired output in a child with developmental dysphasia. *British Journal of Disorders of Communication, 22,* 37–64.

Chomsky, N. (1981). *Lectures on government and binding.* Dordrecht, the Netherlands: Foris.

Clahsen, H. (1989). The grammatical characterization of developmental dysphasia. *Linguistics, 27,* 897–920.

Clahsen, H. (1991). *Child language and developmental dysphasia.* Philadelphia: John Benjamins.

Conti-Ramsden, G. (1990). Maternal recasts and other contingent replies to language-impaired children. *Journal of Speech and Hearing Disorders, 55,* 262–274.

Cramblit, N., & Siegel, G. (1977). The verbal environment of a language-impaired child. *Journal of Speech and Hearing Disorders, 42,* 474–482.

Cross, T.G., Nienhuys, T.G., & Kirkman, M. (1985). Parent–child interaction with receptively disabled children: Some determinants of maternal speech style. In K.E. Nelson (Ed.), *Children's language* (Vol. 5, pp. 247–290). New York: Gardner Press.

Curtiss, S., Katz, W., & Tallal, P. (1992). Delay versus deviance in the language acquisition of language-impaired children. *Journal of Speech and Hearing Research, 35,* 373–383.

Curtiss, S., & Yamada, J. (1988). *The Curtiss-Yamada Comprehensive Language Evaluation (CYCLE).* Unpublished test, University of California, Los Angeles.

Dale, P.S., & Cole, K.N. (1991). What's normal? Specific language impairment in an individual differences perspective. *Language, Speech and Hearing Services in the Schools, 22,* 80–83.

Fletcher, P. (1993, May). *Characterising grammatical impairment: Hope and illusion.* Paper presented at the Symposium for Research in Child Language Disorders, University of Wisconsin, Madison.

Fletcher, P., & Peters, J. (1984). Characterizing language impairment in children: An exploratory study. *Language Testing, 1,* 33–49.

Gertner, B. (1993). *Who do you want to play with? The influence of communicative competence on peer preferences.* Unpublished master's thesis, Department of Speech-Language-Hearing, University of Kansas, Lawrence, KS.

Gopnik, M. (1990a). Feature-blind grammar and dysphasia. *Nature, 344,* 715.

Gopnik, M. (1990b). Feature blindness: A case study. *Language Acquisition, 1,* 139–164.

Gopnik, M., & Crago, M.B. (1991). Familial aggregation of a developmental language disorder. *Cognition, 39,* 1–50.

Hadley, P.A., & Rice, M.L. (1991). Conversational responsiveness of speech and language-impaired preschoolers. *Journal of Speech and Hearing Research, 34,* 1308–1317.

Johnston, J.R. (1988). Specific language disorders in the child. In N. Lass, J. Northern, L. McReynolds, & D.E. Yoder (Eds.), *Handbook of speech-language pathology and audiology* (pp. 685–715). Philadelphia: B.C. Decker.

Johnston, J.R. (1991a). Questions about cognition in children with specific language impairment. In J.F. Miller (Ed.), *Research on child language disorders* (pp. 299–307). Austin, TX: PRO-ED.

Johnston, J.R. (1991b). The continuing relevance of cause: A reply to Leonard's "Specific language impairment as a clinical category." *Language, Speech and Hearing Services in the Schools, 22,* 75–79.

Johnston, J.R., & Kamhi, A.G. (1984). Syntactic and semantic aspects of the utterances of language-impaired children: The same can be less. *Merrill-Palmer Quarterly, 30,* 65–85.

Johnston, J.R., & Smith, L.B. (1989). Dimensional thinking in language-impaired children. *Journal of Speech and Hearing Research, 32,* 33–38.

Kamhi, A.G., & Catts, H.W. (1986). Toward an understanding of developmental language and reading disorders. *Journal of Speech and Hearing Disorders, 51,* 337–347.

Kamhi, A.G., & Catts, H.W. (1989). *Reading disabilities: A developmental language perspective.* New York: Allyn & Bacon.

Khan, L., & James, S. (1983). Grammatical morpheme development in three language disordered children. *Journal of Childhood Communication Disorders, 6,* 85–100.

Lahey, M. (1990). Who shall be called language disordered? Some reflections and one perspective. *Journal of Speech and Hearing Disorders, 55,* 612–620.

Lahey, M., Liebergott, J., Chesnick, M., Menyuk, P., & Adams, J. (1992). Variability in children's use of grammatical morphemes. *Applied Psycholingustics, 13,* 373–398.

Lasky, E., & Klopp, K. (1982). Parent-child interactions in normal and language-disordered children. *Journal of Speech and Hearing Disorders, 47,* 7–18.

Lederberg, A. (1980). The language environment of children with language delays. *Journal of Pediatric Psychology, 5,* 141–159.

Leonard, L.B. (1972). What is deviant language? *Journal of Speech and Hearing Disorders, 37,* 427–446.

Leonard, L.B. (1979). Language impairment in children. *Merrill-Palmer Quarterly, 25,* 205–232.

Leonard, L.B. (1987). Is specific language impairment a useful construct? In S. Rosenberg (Ed.), *Advances in applied psycholinguistics: Disorders of first-language development* (Vol. 1, pp. 1–39). New York: Cambridge University Press.

Leonard, L.B. (1988). Lexical development and processing in specific language impairment. In R.L. Schiefelbusch & L.L. Lloyd (Eds.), *Language perspectives: Acquisition, retardation, and intervention* (2nd ed., pp. 69–87). Austin, TX: PRO-ED.

Leonard, L.B. (1989). Language learnability and specific language impairment in children. *Applied Psycholinguistics, 10,* 179–202.

Leonard, L.B. (1991). Specific language impairment as a clinical category. *Language, Speech and Hearing Services in the Schools, 22,* 66–68.

Leonard, L.B., Bortolini, U., Caselli, M.C., McGregor, K.K., & Sabbadini, L. (1992). Morphological deficits in children with specific language impairment: The status of features in the underlying grammar. *Language Acquisition, 2,* 151–179.

Leonard, L.B., Sabbadini, L., Volterra, V., & Leonard, J.S. (1988). Some influences on the grammar of English- and Italian-speaking children with specific language impairment. *Applied Psycholinguistics, 9,* 39–57.

Lewis, B.A. (1990). Familial phonological disorders: Four pedigrees. *Journal of Speech and Hearing Disorders, 55,* 160–170.

Lewis, B.A. (1993, May). *Genetic considerations in phonological disorders.* Paper presented at the Symposium for Research in Child Language Disorders, University of Wisconsin, Madison, WI.

Lewis, B.A., Ekelman, B.L., & Aram, D.M. (1989). A familial study of severe phonological disorders. *Journal of Speech and Hearing Research, 32,* 713–724.

Ludlow, C.L., & Cooper, J.A. (Eds.). (1983). *Genetic aspects of speech and language disorders.* New York: Academic Press.

Neils, J., & Aram, D.M. (1986). Family history of children with developmental language disorders. *Perceptual and Motor Skills, 63,* 655–658.

Nelson, L.K., Kamhi, A.G., & Apel, K. (1987). Cognitive strengths and weaknesses in language-impaired children: One more look. *Journal of Speech and Hearing Disorders, 52,* 36–43.

Parlour, S. (1990). *Familial risk for articulation disorder: A 28-year follow-up.* Unpublished doctoral dissertation, University of Minnesota, Minneapolis, MN.

Pennington, B.F. (1989). Using genetics to understand dyslexia. *Annals of Dyslexia, 39,* 81–93.

Pinker, S. (1984). *Language learnability and language development.* Cambridge, MA: Harvard University Press.

Pinker, S. (1989a). Resolving a learnability paradox: The acquisition of the verb lexicon. In M.L. Rice & R.L. Schiefelbusch (Eds.), *The teachability of language* (pp. 13–62). Baltimore: Paul H. Brookes Publishing Co.

Pinker, S. (1989b). *Learnability and cognition: The acquisition of argument structure.* Cambridge: Harvard University Press.

Plante, E. (1991). MRI findings in the parents and siblings of specifically language-impaired boys. *Brain and Language, 41,* 67–80.

Plante, E., Swisher, L., Vance, R., & Rapcsak, S. (1991). MRI findings in boys with specific language impairment. *Brain and Language, 41,* 52–66.

Rapin, I., & Allen, D. (1983). Developmental language disorders: Nosologic considerations. In U. Kirk (Ed.), *Neuropsychology of language, reading, and spelling* (pp. 155–184). New York: Academic Press.

Rice, M.L. (1991). Children with specific language impairment: Toward a model of teachability. In N. Krasnegor, D.M. Rumbaugh, R.L. Schiefelbusch, & M. Studdert-Kennedy (Eds.), *Biological and behavioral determinants of language development* (pp. 447–480). Hillsdale, NJ: Lawrence Erlbaum Associates.

Rice, M.L. (1993). "Don't talk to him: He's weird": The role of language in early social interactions. In A.P. Kaiser & D.B. Gray (Eds.), *Enhancing children's communication: Research foundations for intervention* (pp. 139–158). Baltimore: Paul H. Brookes Publishing Co.

Rice, M.L., & Bode, J.V. (1993). GAPS in the verb lexicons of children with specific language impairment. *First Language, 13,* 113–131.

Rice, M.L., Hadley, P.A., & Alexander, A.L. (in press). Social biases toward children with language impairments: A correlative causal model of language limitations. *Applied Psycholinguistics.*

Rice, M.L., & Oetting, J.B. (1993). Morphological deficits of children with SLI: Evaluation of number marking and agreement. *Journal of Speech and Hearing Research, 36,* 1249–1257.

Rice, M.L., Sell, M.A., & Hadley, P.A. (1991). Social interactions of speech and language impaired children. *Journal of Speech and Hearing Research, 34,* 1299–1307.

Stark, R.E., & Tallal, P. (1981). Selection of children with specific language deficits. *Journal of Speech and Hearing Disorders, 46,* 114–122.

Steckol, K., & Leonard, L.B. (1979). The use of grammatical morphemes by normal and language-impaired children. *Journal of Communication Disorders, 12,* 291–301.

Tallal, P. (1976). Rapid auditory processing in normal and disordered language development. *Journal of Speech and Hearing Research, 19,* 561–571.

Tallal, P., & Piercy, M. (1973). Defects of nonverbal auditory perception in children with developmental aphasia. *Nature, 241,* 468–469.

Tallal, P., Ross, P., & Curtiss, S. (1989). Familial aggregation in specific language impairment. *Journal of Speech and Hearing Research, 54,* 167–173.

Tallal, P., Stark, R., Kallman, C., & Mellits, D. (1981). A re-examination of some nonverbal perceptual abilities of language-impaired and normal children as a function of age and sensory modality. *Journal of Speech and Hearing Research, 24,* 351–357.

Tallal, P., Townsend, J., Curtiss, S., & Wulfeck, B. (1991). Phenotypic profiles of language-impaired children based on genetic/family history. *Brain and Language, 41,* 81–95.

Terrell, B.Y., Schwartz, R.G., Prelock, P.A., & Messick, C.K. (1984). Symbolic play in normal and language-impaired children. *Journal of Speech and Hearing Research, 27,* 424–429.

Tomblin, J.B. (1989). Familial concentration of developmental language impairment. *Journal of Speech and Hearing Disorders, 54,* 287–295.

Tomblin, J.B. (1991). Examining the cause of specific language impairment. *Language, Speech and Hearing Services in the Schools, 22,* 69–74.

Tomblin, J.B., Freese, P.R., & Records, N.L. (1990, June). *Language, cognition, and social characteristics of young adults with histories of developmental language disorders.* Paper presented at the Symposium for Research on Child Language Disorders, University of Wisconsin, Madison, WI.

Tomblin, J.B., Freese, P.R., & Records, N.L. (1992). Diagnosing specific language impairment in adults for the purpose of pedigree analysis. *Journal of Speech and Hearing Research, 35,* 832–843.

Wallach, G., & Butler, K. (1984). *Language learning disabilities in school-age children*. Baltimore: Williams & Wilkins.

Wallach, G., & Miller, L. (1988). *Language intervention and academic success*. San Diego: College-Hill.

Watkins, R.V., Buhr, J.C., & Davis, C. (1993, May). *Morphological acquisition in children with language impairments: Evaluation of one derivational form*. Paper presented at the Symposium for Research in Child Language Disorders, University of Wisconsin, Madison, WI.

Watkins, R.V., & Rice, M.L. (1991). Verb particle and preposition acquisition in language-impaired preschoolers. *Journal of Speech and Hearing Research, 34*, 1130–1141.

Watkins, R.V., Rice, M.L., & Moltz, C.C. (1993). Verb use by language-impaired and normally developing children. *First Language, 13*, 133–143.

Wilson, B.C., & Risucci, D.A. (1986). A model for clinical quantification classification. Generation I: Application to language-disordered preschool children. *Brain and Language, 27*, 281–309.

2

Studies of Genetics of Specific Language Impairment

J. Bruce Tomblin and Paula R. Buckwalter

AMONG CHILDREN WITH DEVELOPMENTAL LANGUAGE impairment are some for whom we have no explanation for such an impairment. These children have sufficient hearing for successful language development, normal nonverbal intellectual function as measured by standardized intelligence tests, and they have received what seems to be adequate exposure to language from adult caregivers. In recent years, the term *specific language impairment* (SLI) has been used to refer to this group. During the past 5 years, we have attempted to learn more about the etiology of SLI through studies using methods of genetic epidemiology.

Genetic epidemiology is concerned with the role of genetic mechanisms and their interactions with environmental factors in the etiology of familial diseases. Epidemiology has traditionally been concerned with environmental causes of disease; therefore, the approaches used in genetic epidemiology recognize that genetic expression usually depends on environmental factors. Thus, genetic explanations alone are likely to be insufficient to the understanding of many familial diseases. In order to accomplish this goal, an array of research methods and analytic approaches has been assembled to distinguish among various modes of familial transmission. The most common methods of genetic epidemiology have been pedigree or family studies, twin studies, and adoption studies. In these studies, families or family members are selected because one member, the proband, is known to have the trait or disease of interest. Once a family is selected, relatives of the proband are studied with respect to this trait (phenotype), and a pedigree for each family is constructed. Estimates can then be made of the extent to which the phenotype is genetically determined and/or environmentally determined. Furthermore, if genetic factors are found to contribute to the phenotype, the nature of this

This study was supported by a grant from the National Institutes of Health (NIH USPHS R01 DC00612-02).

genetic mechanism can be inferred from the data contained in the pedigree. In recent years, these methods have been complemented by designs that exploit advances in molecular genetics by obtaining specific information about highly variable sequences of DNA that have known locations on the chromosomes. This genomic information can then be associated with information concerning the phenotypic status of family members to determine the existence and location of genes for the phenotype of interest. Genetic epidemiological studies have begun to provide valuable insights into such complex disorders as schizophrenia, manic-depression (Risch, 1990), alcoholism (Cloninger, 1990), and dyslexia (Pennington, Gilger, Pauls, Smith, Smith, & DeFries, 1991).

FAMILIAL AGGREGATION OF SPECIFIC LANGUAGE IMPAIRMENT

As noted above, genetic epidemiologic research is concerned with the study of diseases with a familial character; thus, if we are to employ this research approach, we must first establish that SLI aggregates in families. If we find that it does, we can narrow the range of possible causal factors to those things that are shared among family members, specifically genes and the environment. Progress toward an understanding of the possible etiology(ies) of SLI has been made recently as a result of replicated evidence that SLI and associated learning problems are concentrated in families. Using a mixture of direct assessment and/or historical reports Neils and Aram (1986), Tallal, Ross, and Curtiss (1989), Tomblin (1989), and Whitehurst, Arnold, Smith, Fischel, Lonigan, and Valdez-Menchaca (1991) have all reported that the immediate relatives of children with SLI had a heightened rate of language and language-related difficulties, as compared to the immediate family members of probands who were typical language learners. Figure 1 summarizes the results of these studies. We can see that three out of four of these studies clearly demonstrate that the rate of language impairment in the relatives of the SLI proband is higher than in the relatives of the non-SLI probands. In these three studies, the average percentage of affected family members of the SLI proband families was 20%, whereas it was 3% in the families of the control probands.

The study of Whitehurst, Arnold, et al. (1991) in Figure 1 does not support a hypothesis of familiality. The probands with language impairment in this study were 2- to 3-year-olds who presented poor expressive vocabulary skills despite normal receptive vocabulary, and the control probands were of similar age without delays in expressive vocabulary development. The phenotype in this study was a parental report of a history of late talking, speech problems, or school problems in the immediate and extended family members. As the authors of this study noted, the children with language impairments were somewhat different from those in the studies that did find a familial pattern. Specifically, these children had impairments that involved

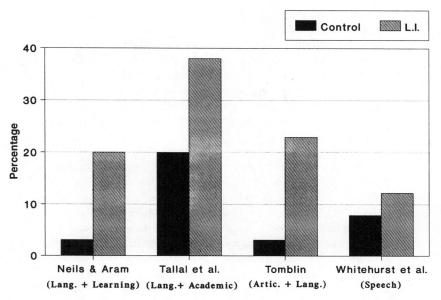

Figure 1. Proportion of first-degree family members determined to have a language impairment in four studies.

expressive language only. Furthermore, in another paper, Whitehurst, Fischel, et al. (1991) also have reported that most of these children did not continue to present these expressive language problems when they were evaluated later at the age of 4 or 5 years. Thus, these children may be viewed as having rather mild language delays that may have been transient rather than persistent. In the other studies the probands were all at least 4 years old and were probably children with more persistent and severe language impairments.

A common feature of all studies on the familiality of SLI is that the authors used historical report for their determination of a language impairment in the adult family members, and some also used this method with the siblings. Moreover, this historical report was usually obtained from one family member. This method may have led to under-reporting of language impairment because adult family members may not have been aware of whether they had had language problems as a child; furthermore, the informant may not have been aware of a positive history of language impairment in another relative. It is also possible to have a differential reporting bias between SLI families and control families so that the parents of children with SLI may have been inclined to report a positive history of language and learning problems because they were led by their child's diagnosis to review their backgrounds as well as those of their family members. In contrast, the parents of the control probands may not have been led to think about their family history.

Thus, it could be claimed that the increased rate of family history in the families with SLI probands was due to this reporting bias.

In order to overcome these problems with studies using historical report, we need family studies of SLI that involve direct assessment of all family members. Recently, Gopnik and Crago (1991) have reported such data in one extended family. In this family, particular difficulty with the use of morphological rules was found in 53% of the family members. Gopnik and Crago have interpreted these results as suggestive of a genetically based deficit of grammatical acquisition.

For the past year and a half we have been conducting a family study of SLI in which we have directly tested all the first-degree family members of SLI probands and often tested extended family members as well. Specifically, our diagnosis of SLI required that the person have normal hearing and a performance IQ of greater than 80. In addition, the children between 3 and 16 were required to have composite language scores 1 standard deviation below the mean for their ages. The language tests used to obtain this composite score varied over this age range, but always included receptive vocabulary and sentence comprehension, as well as measures of expressive grammar.

One challenge for us in doing direct diagnostic testing of family members was the lack of a system for diagnosing SLI in adults. Few, if any, clinicians provide clinical services to adults with SLI; therefore, we could not ask clinicians to provide us with diagnostic standards for the adult with SLI. Furthermore, we were not sure what behavioral domains might continue to reveal SLI in adults. Therefore, before beginning our family studies, we evaluated the performance of 35 young adults with very clear histories of SLI during childhood, and compared their performance to a group of similar young adults lacking such a history (Tomblin, Freese, & Records, 1992). Using a discriminant analysis, we determined which were the most sensitive measures of language impairment. Also, we obtained a discriminant function that predicted the probability of a person's having a language impairment given scores on these measures. Currently, we have been using the probability level of .5 or greater of language impairment to determine language impairment in the adults of our study. Thus, an adult is assigned the SLI phenotype if he or she has a probability level for language impairment of .5 or greater, has normal hearing, and a performance IQ based on the WAIS-R of greater than 80. Those adults for whom English is not their first language or who have acquired aphasia are not included in the SLI phenotype.

Results of Direct Testing

Having established a phenotype for SLI that extends over an age range of 3–70 years, we have now been able to study the occurrence of SLI in the relatives of SLI probands, based upon direct testing rather than historical report. At this point, we have studied 26 families. Table 1 displays the rate of

Table 1.   Rates of SLI in family members of SLI probands when diagnosis was based upon direct assessment

Relationship to proband	Proportion with SLI
Mother	0.15
Father	0.40
Sister	0.06
Brother	0.24

SLI in the first-degree family members. The overall rate of SLI in these family members was 21%. We have no control families because this study focused on pedigrees of SLI families only. However, the overall rate of SLI in these families is very similar to the rates obtained in the prior studies using family history, and it is very unlikely that we would find rates close to these levels in the general population. Adding to the credibility of these data is the strong pattern for SLI to occur more frequently in males than females. These data support the conclusion that SLI has a strong familial quality and demonstrate that familiality reported in prior studies is not likely to be influenced by a reporting bias.

The rate of 21% is not necessarily an accurate representation of the proportion of affected family members in all these families because 58% of the SLI probands were isolates. That is, they had no other affected first-degree family member. This also means that in those probands with other affected family members, we often found several affected members. Tallal, Townsend, Curtiss, and Wulfeck (1991) also found this pattern of heavy concentration of SLI in some families and then a high rate of isolated cases. Because there seem to be two types of SLI probands—those with other SLI relatives and those without such relatives—we need to begin to consider whether this represents two different groups with two different etiologies. Tallal et al. have performed a preliminary inquiry into this issue and found little to differentiate the familial and nonfamilial groups. If, in fact, the two groups do not differ with respect to etiology and if there is a genetic basis for SLI in the familial group, then we would have to consider the possibility that SLI does not always occur, even when an individual has the SLI genotype. Therefore, there are family members with the genetic predisposition for SLI, but who do not show signs of it. Such a pattern is termed *incomplete penetrance,* where penetrance represents the proportion of individuals with the genotype who present the phenotype. Incomplete penetrance of SLI would suggest that such factors as the environment or other genes influence whether a person with the genetic predisposition for SLI will, in fact, have SLI. At this time, the occurrence of a high rate of isolated cases of SLI could mean that either we have etiologic heterogeneity for SLI, or that the genetic basis for SLI is incompletely penetrant.

By combining the research using family history data and the evidence from family studies in which family members have been directly assessed, it seems clear that SLI has a strong familial character. The research questions now must focus on learning what factors contribute to this familiality. Specifically, we must ask to what extent this condition is the product of genetic factors, the biologic environment of the fetus and infant, or the linguistic environment. As noted earlier, genetic epidemiology is well suited to addressing questions of this sort by providing methods for testing different modes of familial inheritance.

EVIDENCE OF A GENETIC BASIS FOR SLI FAMILIALITY

Once a trait is found to have a familial character, the natural question is whether this familial pattern is due, at least in part, to genes shared among the family members and/or if this pattern is the result of the environment shared by family members. Often, early evidence addressing this comes from twin studies. Twins provide a very convenient natural experiment for genetic research. Identical (monozygotic, MZ) twins are genetic clones of each other; thus, they share all their genes. Fraternal (dizygotic, DZ) twins share only 50% of their genes; thus, they are genetically the same as any other sibling relationship. The two types of twins, however, do not differ with respect to their environment, or at least this assumption is made in twin research. If a condition is genetically influenced, we should expect to find that the MZ twins are more similar (concordant) to each other, with respect to the trait, than are the DZ twins because the MZ twins share more genes than the DZ twins.

Oddly, there have been no extensive twin studies of children with SLI. There have been some case reports of SLI in twins, but little can be made of these because we need a much larger number of twins before we can perform the necessary statistical tests. A few years ago, we performed a simple twin pilot study. A questionnaire was sent to a large number of public school speech-language clinicians in Iowa asking if they had twins in their caseload. If they did, we asked them to report the speech and language status of each twin, as well as the educational status, sex, and type of twinship. Those children identified as having a language impairment, but not identified as mentally retarded or hearing impaired, we considered as SLI in this study. We found that of 82 twin pairs (56 MZ and 26 same sex DZ) 38% of the DZ were concordant for SLI, and 80% of the MZ twins were concordant. Thus, those twins who shared all their genes were much more likely to be similar with respect to SLI than the DZ.

Zygosity, that is, whether the twinship was DZ or MZ, in this study was based only on the report of the clinician; thus, it cannot be viewed as a very refined measure. The data from this study, therefore, must be viewed with caution. Lewis and Thompson (1991), using a better measure of zygosity, have reported similar values of concordance for a group of twins with specific language and phonological disorders. Recognizing that the ideal SLI twin study has not been done yet, we can use the data from these studies to suggest that there is the possibility of substantial genetic contribution to SLI. If this is true, we then need to question the nature of this genetic transmission among family members.

MODES OF FAMILIAL INHERITANCE

Multifactorial/Polygenic Mode

People differ from one another in such familial traits as stature, skin color, and intelligence in a gradual or continuous fashion. We usually can measure these traits in a quantitative manner, demonstrating that people have more or less of the trait. Moreover, the values of these measures will often approximate the normal distribution in large diverse populations. Such quantitative traits as these are usually the result of several causal factors, each contributing a little to a person's obtained level for the trait. Thus, a person's height is determined by more than one gene; furthermore, it is influenced by such factors as childhood health and diet. When a trait is the result of many factors it is described as a *multifactorial trait*.

Leonard (1987) has proposed that children with SLI are not qualitatively different than language learners without impairments, but rather they may be viewed as simply less adept in language learning than the majority of the population. Furthermore, he noted that the same factors that contribute to individual differences among children without SLI also contribute to the variance differentiating children with SLI from children without SLI and that there is no special causal factor contributing to SLI. Thus, according to this view, there would not be an SLI gene or a pathogenic environment that would lead to SLI, as would be found in individuals with Down syndrome or language learners deafened by meningitis. His proposal is compatible with a multifactorial account for normal and SLI language development, which would predict that individual differences in language acquisition proficiency are the product of numerous factors all contributing a small amount to the overall level of proficiency for language learners both with and without SLI. If these factors are transmitted in families, a familial aggregation of SLI would occur as a result of certain families carrying several factors that are disadvantageous for language learning.

A Single Major Gene

Some familial traits are not the product of several factors, but are primarily the result of a single gene. These traits usually are not distributed in a continuous fashion among individuals, but they seem to exist as qualitatively different forms. Examples of this mode of inheritance are the A, B, and O blood types or the absence of functional dystrophin in muscle cells in muscular dystrophy and its presence in healthy muscle tissue. When variance in a trait is the product of different forms of a single gene (alleles), the pattern of transmission from parents to offspring can usually be found to fit one of the patterns of single gene transmission described by Mendel, such as dominant or recessive; thus, these traits are referred to as *mendelian*.

Recently Gopnik (1990) and Gopnik and Crago (1991) have argued that SLI may be a very discrete and rather complete inability to acquire certain aspects of language, and that this may be caused by a single gene. Evidence for this claim comes from the study of an extended family in which some family members have difficulty both producing morphological endings on novel word forms and performing metalinguistic judgments of sentences that violate morphological rules. Other members of this family who were not impaired were reported to have acquired morphological rules. Gopnik has proposed that this pattern of competent and incompetent morphological development in close relatives provides evidence of a single gene influencing grammatical disability in these family members with SLI.

Additional support for a mendelian account of SLI comes from recent family studies of developmental dyslexia. Although dyslexia is defined in terms of reading impairment, whereas SLI is defined in terms of oral language impairment, these two conditions are regarded as closely related conditions, if not variants of the same condition. Also, dyslexia runs in families, and recently Pennington et al. (1991) have reported evidence of a single major gene involved in the familial transmission of dyslexia. These authors note that linkage studies of dyslexia using methods of molecular genetics have implicated chromosome 15 as a possible locus for such a gene; however, genetic heterogeneity is possible, with different loci involved for different families.

Mixed Mode

A third mode of familial transmission is a mixture of a single abnormal gene contributing to a substantial portion of the variance of the condition, plus additional variance depending on multifactorial causes involving other genes or environmental factors. This mode of transmission is often described as a *mixed model*.

TESTS OF THE MODE OF TRANSMISSION FOR SLI

With these models as possible hypotheses of the mode of familial transmission of SLI, we can begin to examine some data that address these hypotheses and methods for testing which of these models is most likely.

Commingling Analysis

Recall that in the multifactorial mode of transmission, many genetic and environmental factors come together to produce a complex quantitative trait with a normal distribution that can be described best with one mean. In contrast, a quantitative trait with a single locus will generate a multimodal distribution that requires several means, each characterizing a different sub-population. If data concerning some quantitative trait are available from a large, unbiased sample of people, it should be possible to use these data to see if the distribution conforms to a multifactorial trait or a single locus trait.

Commingling is an analytic technique developed to do this. Specifically, commingling analysis attempts to fit obtained data to various hypothetical distributions involving one or more means, and tests these fits using maximum likelihood methods. Models with additional parameters, that is, more means and standard deviations, are selected only if they are found to fit the data better. Thus, the objective is to find the simplest model that accounts for the greatest amount of the variance in the obtained data.

This approach has been used to determine the role of genetic and environmental factors in obesity (Moll, Burns, & Lauer, 1991). The dependent variable was a body mass index, which is the ratio of weight to height. In this study, the best fit was obtained with two means or subcomponents, as shown in Figure 2. This analysis provided some evidence, then, that a causal mechanism functioning as a single gene resulted in two distributions—one for those with average weight/height ratios and a second for those who are heavier than would be expected for their height. We should note that each distribution

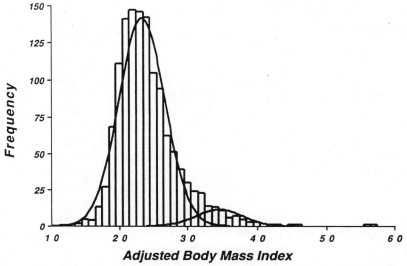

Figure 2. The distribution of adjusted body mass index (vertical bars) with the two distributions fit to the body mass distribution using commingling. (From Moll, P.P., Burns, T.L., & Lauer, R. [1991]. The genetic and environmental sources of body mass index variability: The Muscatine ponderosity family study. *American Journal of Human Genetics, 49,* 1249; reprinted by permission of The University of Chicago Press.)

shows considerable variance and, in fact, there is overlap. Therefore, a single gene alone would be insufficient to account for these data. In this case, the results are consistent with a mixed model in which environmental factors and polygenes account for some of the variance, but in addition, a single recessive genetic locus contributes to a considerable amount of the variance in this distribution of the body mass index.

The example above shows how commingling can be used to determine whether a trait seems to conform to the distributional characteristics of a purely multifactorial trait or to one with a qualitative etiologic basis, such as a single genetic locus. In light of this, we have submitted language data to a commingling analysis. These data were obtained from a large sample (647) of children age 5–7 years who had been administered the Test of Oral Language Development-2:Primary (TOLD-2:P; Newcomer & Hammill, 1988). These children had been participating in a prospective longitudinal study concerned with birth risk factors and language outcome at school age.

The data reflecting the performance of these children on the Grammatic Completion and Picture Vocabulary subtests were used. We chose to analyze these two subtests separately because these two tests reflect language performance in two domains that may represent two different underlying language acquisition mechanisms; an association-based system for vocabulary development and a rule-based system for morphological development (Pinker, 1991). In addition, SLI children seem to find morphological development more challenging than lexical acquisition (Leonard, 1989; Moore & Johnston, 1991; Watkins & Rice, 1991).

Figure 3 shows the distribution of the obtained Picture Identification scale scores of the TOLD-2:P in the form of a frequency histogram. Superimposed over this histogram is a curve representing the results of the commingling analysis. The results suggest that the best model for the obtained data entails one mean and one standard deviation. Thus, these data do not offer any evidence that lexical skill in young children is influenced by a single qualitative factor such as a single gene; rather, these results are consistent with a multifactorial model underlying the acquisition of lexical ability.

Figure 3 also shows the results of the commingling analysis for the Grammatic Completion. In this case, the obtained distribution was best described as being the result of two populations. One subpopulation, with a mean scale score of 10.06, contained 80% of the total group, and another group, with a higher mean of 14.35, comprised 20% of the group. These data are suggestive of some discrete factor underlying performance on this task. Those individuals possessing one value (0) of this trait are likely to be in the lower distribution, whereas, those with the other value of the trait (1) may be in the higher group. These results are consistent with a mixed model of the basis of morphological skill development. Moreover, it seems that different factors are contributing to the distribution of morphological skill development

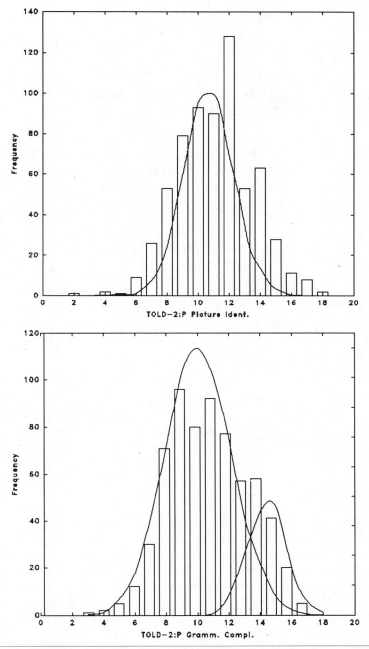

Figure 3.   The upper panel contains the distribution of TOLD-2:P picture identification standard scores with a one-component distribution fit to the data using commingling analysis. The lower panel presents the distribution of TOLD-2:P grammatical completion standard scores with two-component distributions fitted to the data using commingling analysis.

than for vocabulary development, thus supporting the contention of those making such a claim.

Unfortunately, this analysis did not reveal a group with particularly low grammatical skills that might represent a language-impaired or SLI subpopulation. Two explanations may be proposed to explain the absence of a lower group:

1. Children with SLI, at least with respect to this measure, simply represent the tail of a normal distribution of the trait and, therefore, they do not separate themselves from the remainder of the typical group of children—an account consistent with Leonard's (1987) predictions.

2. It is possible that there were so few SLI children in the sample that they could not be detected. The mean scores of these children were approximately two thirds of a standard deviation higher than that of the normative group for this test. Fewer than 4% fell below the 16th percentile. Clearly, this sample was biased because it contained only the children of parents who remained in one area for the 5–7 years of the longitudinal study; thus, these children came from homes with a higher socioeconomic status. This bias may have reduced the number of children with poor grammatical abilities in our sample to a point that, if a distinctive lower group existed, the commingling analysis could not detect it.

This commingling analysis must be viewed as very preliminary and data from a larger and unbiased sample of children is now needed. The results are somewhat encouraging, however, in that the aspect of language that seems most affected in children with SLI is also the area that shows some evidence of an underlying qualitative trait.

Analysis of Pedigrees

Commingling provides evidence for the presence or absence of separate distributions, which may then suggest that either a mixed model or multifactorial model of transmission contributes to the disorder. Commingling, however, does not provide a direct test for different modes of familial transmission. In order to test for these modes of transmission, it is necessary first to obtain data on the phenotype of interest (SLI in this case) from family members, and then test these data against predictions made by models of different mechanisms of transmission. Thus, it is necessary to construct family pedigrees for SLI and associated conditions, such as reading impairment. These pedigrees may be viewed as a complex system of data having to do with the biologic relationships of family members, the phenotypic status of these family members, and their gender.

We are now engaged in a pedigree study of SLI with the objective of using these data to make inferences about the possible mode(s) of inheritance of SLI. The basic criteria for the SLI phenotype for children and adults were described in the section concerned with familial aggregation. The SLI probands in this study are age 7–10, and were recruited from the caseloads of public school clinicians. Once the family agrees to participate in the study, a researcher visits the home, and by means of an interview with a parent, constructs a pedigree of the proband's family, covering first-, second-, and in the case of cousins, third-degree relatives of the proband. At this time, we ask about family history of speech, language, reading, academic problems, mental retardation, and psychiatric disorders. Also, we ask about autoimmune problems in the first-degree relatives of the proband because there have been reports of an association between autoimmune disease and dyslexia (Pennington, Smith, Kimberling, Green, & Haith, 1987), and Geschwind and Galaburda (1985) have predicted that such an association should also be found for SLI children.

We ask about these associated conditions because we want to determine if SLI and these conditions co-occur in families, even if they do not always co-occur in individuals. In particular, we need to recognize that there is not always a simple 1:1 relationship between a genotype and a phenotype; that is, all persons with a particular single gene disease will not necessarily present this disease in the same degree or the same fashion. As a result, the condition may have variable expression in that the degree or form of the trait may vary across individuals with the same genetic background for the trait. If there is a genetic basis for SLI, we must consider the possibility that SLI is only one form of a broader condition that may involve dyslexia and phonological impairment, or other language-learning disorders. Different individuals in the family may show different patterns of learning difficulties, and as a result, an analysis of the pedigrees only for SLI could fail to detect a pattern of genetic transmission.

At this time, we have completed pedigrees for 26 families containing an average of 38.6 members each, or 1,004 people. To perform a diagnostic test on all these family members would require a substantial amount of time. However, we can reduce this by using a method of sampling in the families called *sequential sampling,* and we do not test all members of an extended family. The rule for sequential sampling is that all first-degree relatives of affected family members are tested. Thus, we automatically test all first-degree relatives of the proband. If a parent is identified as affected, then we will test all the first-degree relatives of this parent. This sampling technique has been found to be as powerful as a complete sampling method, and it reduces the number of persons we need to test (Boehnke, Young, & Moll, 1988).

General prevalence data for SLI in the immediate family members of these 26 probands were presented earlier. The data contained in the pedigrees from these families can be used to test various hypotheses about the transmission of SLI using various methods.

One simple method was proposed by Penrose (1953). With this method, the mode of genetic transmission of diseases can be evaluated simply by knowing the rate of the disease in siblings of probands and the rate in the general population. From our study, we know the rate of SLI in brothers and sisters of SLI probands. We are not as sure about the rate of SLI in the general population; however, if we assume that the prevalence of SLI in males is 0.06 and females is 0.02, we can compute the relative frequency of SLI in the siblings of the SLI probands in our study, and compare this value with the predicted relative frequency for the major modes of inheritance, namely a dominant single gene, a recessive single gene, or a multifactorial pattern. These data are presented in Table 2. We can see that the closest fit between the obtained (s/q) and expected values is the multifactorial model, which has an expected relative frequency for males of 4.08 and 7.07 for females. These results suggest that our SLI phenotype is the product of several factors, such as several genetic loci and/or several environmental factors. We must caution that these results are merely suggestive of a multifactorial mode of transmission. A limitation of Penrose's procedure is that it does not provide a means of testing the goodness of fit between the obtained and expected values. We can see, for instance, in Table 2 that the obtained value for females (3.0) is not very close to the expected value of 7.07, but we cannot determine whether this is a good fit or a poor fit.

Complex Segregation Analysis

Since the early 1970s, a powerful method, complex segregation analysis, has become the standard tool of genetic epidemiology. This statistical method provides tests for various modes of transmission of a trait among related individuals. This is a very complex, computer-based analytic method, and space does not permit a complete description of this procedure. Several different computer-based approaches to segregation analysis exist. We are currently using the program *Pedigree Analysis Package* (PAP) (Hasstedt, 1989). In very

Table 2. A comparison between obtained relative frequency of SLI and relative frequencies expected based upon dominant recessive and multifactorial modes of inheritance

Obtained				Expected		
General population	Siblings			Dominant	Recessive	Multifactorial
(q)	(s)	(s/q)		$(1/2q)$	$(1/4q)$	$(1/\sqrt{q})$
Males	0.06	0.24	4	8.33	4.16	4.08
Females	0.02	0.06	3	25.00	12.15	7.07

Relative frequency (s/q) is computed by dividing the prevalence of SLI in siblings of SLI probands (s) by the prevalence of SLI in the general population (q). This obtained relative frequency can be compared to the expected values for each mode of genetic transmission. The coefficients for each mode (1/2, 1/4, $1/\sqrt{\ }$) represent the probability of a sibling being affected given an affected proband. The expected rate for each mode then is the product of the prevalence rate in the general population multiplied by the coefficient for the particular mode.

simple terms, complex segregation analysis involves fitting obtained phenotypic data of family members to probabilities of family members having certain gene types (alleles), as predicted by various models of genetic transmission. The segregation analysis method provides a goodness of fit test for different modes of transmission.

The first step in the analysis is to fit the data to a general model of transmission. This model contains all the parameters concerned with transmission (nine in this case). In the general model, all parameters are unconstrained; that is, they are not required to conform to any particular mode of transmission. The analysis package attempts to arrive at values for these parameters that best fit the data based on maximum likelihood estimates. This model then serves as a baseline against which other models of specific transmission are tested. In these more constrained models, the parameters, particularly the transmission parameters, are fixed, and the results are compared with the "best fit" data obtained from the general model.

At this stage, we have been unable to obtain a solution for the general model using our SLI phenotype. Therefore, we cannot proceed to test the more specific models. In particular, we haven't been able to arrive at an accurate estimate of an allele frequency for SLI. It is likely that the main reason we have not arrived at a solution is that we have too few families and, therefore, we must continue to gather more data. Segregation analysis requires several pedigrees in order to have the power to test the various models. Based on estimates of SLI prevalence and recurrence rates in families, we may need to obtain data on 75 extended families.

We have to consider at this point, however, that there are other reasons for our unsuccessful early attempts at segregation analysis. Segregation analysis makes inferences about the possible genetic mechanisms involved in a disease, based on the phenotypic data entered in the pedigree. If there are genetic factors that are involved in the etiology of SLI, but these factors are expressed in a phenotype that differs from ours, then the segregation analysis would fail to reveal these genetic factors. Thus, in addition to our sample size, we must consider whether an alternate phenotype is needed.

Our phenotype is based on clinical standards and clinical measures. We can not be sure that all those who are diagnosed by these standards have the same etiology. It could be very possible that those individuals identified with SLI using our scheme are etiologically heterogeneous. Thus, one alternate phenotype would be a diagnostic category that is more restrictive, and thus, also more likely to be etiologically homogeneous. Gopnik and Crago's (1991) phenotype exemplifies such a more limited phenotype because they focus only on the grammatical rule deficits in their work.

Narrowing the scope of the diagnostic category assumes that the putative genetic basis for SLI affects a very specific language domain. We must also consider the possibility that our current SLI phenotype is already too narrow. There is considerable evidence of a strong association between SLI and reading difficulties (Aram & Hall, 1989; Kamhi & Catts, 1986). It is possible that all these language-learning problems have the same genetic basis, but we are confronted with variable expression of this genetic factor. Hence, in some individuals, the gene(s) is (are) expressed as a reading problem, whereas in others it is expressed as a spoken language impairment.

We are now in the process of constructing both broader and narrower phenotypes, using the data we have obtained from our families. We will evaluate these redefined phenotypes using complex segregation analysis. Clearly, at this time, we are in an exploratory phase of our genetic epidemiologic studies of SLI. It is unlikely that our first efforts will yield straightforward answers about a condition as complex as SLI.

Fortunately, our field is not alone in attempting to understand a complex familial disorder. Recently, Rice and Risch (1989) noted, with respect to the genetic epidemiologic study of affective disorders (manic depression, depression, cyclothymia, etc.), that:

> the affective disorders may be a genetic epidemiologist's nightmare. There are age and sex effects . . . . There is considerable phenotypic heterogeneity . . . and genetic heterogeneity. There is a lack of "gold standard" for diagnosis and no clear consensus on who should be classified as a case—especially for milder forms of the affective disorders . . . . However, these complexities are not unique to the affective disorders . . . .
>
> In many respects, the complexities involved in genetic analysis of affective disorders are common to many genetically complex diseases, and methodological conclusions can be generally applicable. (p. 165)

The same situation holds for language-learning disorders encompassing SLI and reading impairment, as well as for other forms of developmental language impairment. We cannot assume that answers concerning the familial basis of SLI will come quickly or easily. Fortunately, as Rice and Risch (1989) suggest, developments in allied fields, such as psychiatry, may provide us with useful methods for resolving these difficult challenges.

CONCLUSIONS

The data we have seen so far provide clear evidence, based on a standard diagnostic protocol, that SLI does run in families. The twin data, although limited, provide support for the belief that a substantial portion of this familial pattern is likely to have genetic causes. Finally, it is still too early to determine what the nature of this genetic cause is. Our very preliminary data support a multifactorial/polygenic mode, but we need to study more families and to consider alternative phenotypes before we can arrive at solid conclusions.

REFERENCES

Aram, D., & Hall, N. (1989). Longitudinal follow-up of children with preschool communication disorders: Treatment implications. *School Psychology Review, 18,* 487–501.

Boehnke, M., Young, M., & Moll, P. (1988). Comparison of sequential and fixed-structure sampling of pedigrees in complex segregation analysis of a quantitative trait. *American Journal of Human Genetics, 43,* 336–343.

Cloninger, C.R. (1990). Genetic epidemiology of alcoholism: Observations critical in the design and analysis of linkage studies. In C.R. Cloninger & H. Begleiter (Eds.), *Genetics and biology of alcoholism* (pp. 105-129). Cold Spring Harbor, NY: Cold Spring Harbor Laboratory.

Geschwind, N., & Galaburda, A.M. (1985). Cerebral lateralization. Biological mechanisms, associations, and pathology: I. *Archives of Neurology, 42,* 428–459.

Gopnik, M. (1990). Feature-blind grammar and dysphasia. *Nature, 344,* 715.

Gopnik, M., & Crago, M.B. (1991). Familial aggregation of a developmental language disorder. *Cognition, 39,* 1–50.

Hasstedt, S.J. (1989). Pedigree Analysis Package *Technical Report #13,* Department of Medical Biophysics and Computing, University of Utah, Salt Lake City.

Kamhi, A.G., & Catts, H.W. (1986). Toward an understanding of developmental language and reading disorders. *Journal of Speech and Hearing Disorders, 51,* 337–347.

Leonard, L. (1987). Is specific language impairment a useful construct? In S. Rosenberg (Ed.), *Advances in applied psycholinguistics: Disorders of first-language development* (Vol. I, pp. 1–39). New York: Cambridge University Press.

Leonard, L.B. (1989). Language learnability and specific language impairment in children. *Applied Psycholinguistics, 10,* 179–202.

Lewis, B.A., & Thompson, L. (1991, November). *A twin study of developmental speech and language disorders.* Paper presented at the Annual Convention of the American Speech-Language-Hearing Association, Atlanta, GA.

Moll, P.P., Burns, T.L., & Lauer, R. (1991). The genetic and environmental sources of body mass index variability: The Muscatine ponderosity family study. *American Journal of Human Genetics, 49,* 1243–1255.

Moore, M.E., & Johnston, J.R. (1991, June). *Adverbial and inflectional expressions of past time by normal and language-impaired children.* Paper presented at the Symposium for Research on Child Language Disorders, Madison, WI.

Neils, J., & Aram, D.M. (1986). Family history of children with developmental language disorders. *Perceptual and Motor Skills, 63,* 655–658.

Newcomer, P.L., & Hammill, D.D. (1988). *Test of Oral Language Development-2: Primary.* Austin, TX: PRO-ED.

Pennington, B.F., Gilger, J.W., Pauls, D., Smith, S.A., Smith, S.D., & DeFries, J.C. (1991). Evidence for major gene transmission of developmental dyslexia. *Journal of the American Medical Association, 266,* 1527–1534.

Pennington, B., Smith, S., Kimberling, W., Green, P., & Haith, M. (1987). Left-handedness and immune disorders in familial dyslexics. *Archives of Neurology, 44,* 634–639.

Penrose, L.S. (1953). The genetical background of common diseases. *Acta Genetica, 4,* 257–265.

Pinker, S. (1991). Rules of language. *Science, 253,* 530–535.

Rice, J., & Risch, N. (1989). Genetic analysis of the affective disorders: Summary of GAW5. *Genetic Epidemiology, 6,* 161–177.

Tallal, P., Ross, R., & Curtiss, S. (1989). Familial aggregation in specific language impairment. *Journal of Speech and Hearing Disorders, 54,* 167–173.

Tallal, P., Townsend, J., Curtiss, S., & Wulfeck, B. (1991). Phenotypic profiles of language-impaired children based on genetic/family history. *Brain and Language, 41,* 81–95.

Tomblin, J.B. (1989). Familial concentration of developmental language impairment. *Journal of Speech and Hearing Disorders, 54,* 287–295.

Tomblin, J.B., Freese, P.R., & Records, N.L. (1992). Diagnosing specific language impairment in adults for the purpose of pedigree analysis. *Journal of Speech and Hearing Research, 35,* 832–843.

Watkins, R.V., & Rice, M.L. (1991). Verb particle and preposition acquisition in language-impaired preschoolers. *Journal of Speech and Hearing Research, 34,* 1130–1141.

Whitehurst, G.J., Arnold, D.S., Smith, M., Fischel, J.E., Lonigan, C.J., & Valdez-Menchaca, M.C. (1991). Family history in developmental expressive language delay. *Journal of Speech and Hearing Research, 34,* 1150–1157.

Whitehurst, G.J., Fischel, J.E., Lonigan, C.J., Valdez-Menchaca, M.C., Arnold, D.S., & Smith, M. (1991). Treatment of early expressive language delay; If, when, and how. *Topics in Language Disorders, 11,* 55–68.

3

From Families to Phenotypes

Theoretical and
Clinical Implications of Research into the
Genetic Basis of Specific Language Impairment

Martha B. Crago and Myrna Gopnik

SUBSTANTIVE CLAIMS HAVE BEEN MADE concerning the genetic basis of language and the nature of developmental language impairment based on evidence from a study of a large British family. At the American Academy for the Advancement of Sciences meeting in February 1992, Gopnik reported that:

> . . . there is now empirical evidence that shows that a single dominant gene is associated with the ability to construct symbolic rules in the grammar. These rules have several different consequences in the grammar including agreement of nouns and pronouns, nouns with verbs, and the tense of verbs. . . . This population of genetically language-impaired subjects provides us with a natural experiment that can directly address the fundamental questions as to how much of language is innate and just what aspects are under genetic control. (p. 1)

Following Gopnik's presentation, numerous reports appeared in the press and on the radio about the discovery of a gene for grammar. These reports ranged from accurate reporting (Fitzgerald, 1992) to farfetched humor (Bombeck, 1992), and everything in between. This chapter presents some of the claims made by Gopnik (1992), Gopnik (in press), and Gopnik and Crago (1991), citing evidence for these claims and postulating about further evidence needed to understand more thoroughly the genetic basis for language impairment. In doing so, the family aggregate whose language served as the basis for these claims is described and ramifications of the research findings for the charac-

We thank our wonderful research assistants: Janis Oram, Susan Methe, Lori Hadzipetros, and Shanley Allen. This research was made possible through a generous grant from the Social Sciences and Humanities Research Council of Canada. Our special thanks go to Dr. Patrick Dunne of Baylor University for his advice concerning the genetics issues described in this chapter. Finally, our greatest gratitude goes to the British family we studied for their willingness to help solve the puzzle of their impairment.

terization of specific language impairment (SLI) is discussed. The family aggregate in question has been the focus of study by two distinct research groups (Gopnik & Crago, 1991; Hurst, Baraitser, Auger, Graham,   Norell, 1990; Pembrey, 1992). Our particular research has centered on an examination of this family's language from the standpoint of linguistic theory using a case study approach.

ISSUES IN THE FAMILY CASE STUDY APPROACH

In 1989, Tomblin described epidemiologic evidence for the familial aggregation of SLI and proposed that important additional evidence for the genetic basis of language impairment would be available from the study of a large multigenerational family affected by SLI.

Case study of a large family allows the exclusion of environmental interpretations of SLI by contrasting the affected members of a family with unaffected members of the same family. Indeed, it is highly unlikely that a parent could give grammatically different input to different children, particularly if that parent is affected by language impairment herself. A parent might speak more or differently to certain children, but the form of input to children that would be necessary to produce deficits such as tense marking is not consciously controlled, and, therefore, could not be willfully altered by a parent. The fact that some of the children in large family aggregations whose parents are affected by SLI have developed normal language is perhaps even more striking evidence that an environmental explanation is not sufficient.

Family case studies fall in between individual case studies and studies using small group data. As group studies, they are subject to a variety of naturalistic and other constraints. One hazard is that the number of subjects is large enough to make group comparisons, but small enough that these comparisons are often made on the basis of very few subjects. Furthermore, the subjects in such a study are nonreplaceable, thus subject attrition results in even smaller numbers. The size of the sample and the intersubject variability, then, are important issues to consider in between-group comparisons within such a family case study.

CHARACTERISTICS OF THE LARGE FAMILY AGGREGATE

The language data presented later in this chapter come from a large, three-generational, British family. Of the 30 family members, 16 have been diagnosed as affected with SLI (see Figure 1). Family members range in age from a 4-year-old granddaughter to a 76-year-old grandmother. Intelligence (WISC-R) scores (see Figure 2) are available for only five of the third-generation family members affected by SLI. Four of these scores show verbal performance discrepancies of 18–37 points. The fifth family member's measured IQ score falls just outside the usual cutoff point (performance IQ = 85)

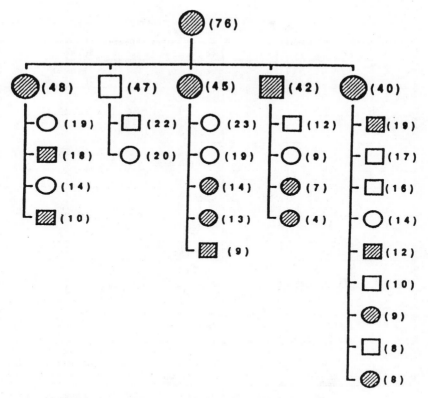

Figure 1. The family. (○ = female subject, □ = male subject, ◍ or ▨ = impaired.)

for SLI. Her verbal and performance scores are only marginally different. However, she clearly is not seriously developmentally delayed. In the second generation of the family, there is one female who is reported by the grandmother to have been a slow learner. The affected male in this generation reported that he has been on medication for schizophrenia for over 20 years. This man also has dysfluencies in his speech. Furthermore, one of the affected members in the third generation, a young man in his 20s, is presently very withdrawn and uncommunicative. This is reportedly a marked change in his behavior over the last 2 years. This young man, as well as certain other family members, have been abused and threatened by their unaffected parents or spouses. Nevertheless, all the other family members we tested were extremely gregarious, sociable, and cooperative.

Several affected members of the family presently have or have had seriously disturbed phonology. They do not, however, have any impairment of the oral peripheral mechanism, either from the point of view of structure or movement, with the exception of dental malocclusion (Gopnik & Crago, in

Dysphasic subjects

Sex	Ages	IQ	School	Work
F	76		regular	nurse's aide
F	48		regular; speech therapy	cleaner
F	45		regular; speech therapy	
M	42		regular; speech therapy	driver
F	40		regular; speech therapy	
M	18		special	chef
M	10	VIQ: 81 PIQ: 82	special	
F	7	VIQ: 79 PIQ: 103	special	
M	19		special	nightwatchman
M	12	VIQ: 72 PIQ: 107	special	
F	9	VIQ: 72 PIQ: 98	special	
F	8	VIQ: 70 PIQ: 107	special	

Normal subjects

Sex	Ages	IQ	School	Work
F	19		normal	clerk/typist
F	14		normal	clerk/typist
F	9		normal	
M	17		normal	
M	16		normal	
F	14		normal	
M	10		normal	
M	8		normal	

Figure 2. Subject characteristics.

press). Repetition of multiple varied syllables (pa/ta/ka) is, however, diffi-cult for affected family members. Similarly, certain members have difficulty sequencing sounds in words. Their error patterns are variable, with some consonant clusters, for example, being simplified (st/str) and others being made more complex (str/st) (Gopnik & Crago, in press).

All family members affected with SLI, except for the grandmother, have had speech and language intervention. Four of the affected members in the second generation attended normal public schools and had supplemental speech and language intervention. The other female from this generation attended a different school, one described by her family as a school for slow learners. The family members with SLI in the third generation attended the Lionel School for Aphasic Children, on the outskirts of London. This is a specialized school for children with language impairment. In British schools such as this, children are screened for entry in order to exclude possible diagnoses of hearing impairment, global developmental delay, and autism. Children attending such schools represent a variety of types of language problems, including severe phonological problems and apraxia.

CONVERGING GENETIC EVIDENCE

Gopnik (1992) and Gopnik and Crago (1991) point out that there is converging evidence from three sources for the genetic basis for SLI. The first is from epidemiological studies of the type that Tomblin and Buckwalter describe in this volume (Chapter 2). His earlier work (Tomblin, 1989) and that of Tallal, Ross, and Curtiss (1989) document the significant difference between the incidence of positive family histories of SLI among first-degree relatives of SLI children and those of the controls. A second source of genetic evidence is twin studies (Borges-Osorio & Salzano, 1985; Lewis & Thompson, 1992; Tomblin, 1991). These studies show that each twin in a monozygotic pair is much more likely to have language impairment than are dyzgotic twins. Slightly different evidence has been reported by Bishop (1992), who found that monozygotic twins were more likely to be affected by moderate levels of SLI, rather than more severe levels of SLI. At the neurological, level, certain effects associated with the genetic disposition for SLI have been reported by Plante (1991) and Plante, Swisher, Vance, and Rapcsak (1991). This research indicates that genetic differences may cause differences at the level of the neural substrate. Plante's research, based on a small number of subjects, indicates that atypical symmetries in the neurological substrate are associated with language impairment. Furthermore, the risk factor for such neurological impairment seems to be transmitted through families. As mentioned at the outset of this chapter, genetic evidence also comes from studies of families with several members affected by SLI. Our work, as is that of Samples and Lane (1985), is based on this form of evidence. Hurst et al. (1990) and Pembrey (1992) claim that the distribution of the family members we have studied is congruent with a pattern of inheritance caused by a single autosomal dominant gene.

Further Genetic Evidence

Other evidence about the nature of genetically based language impairment could be available from a genetic blood analysis. Linkage studies, in which a language gene is linked to a polymorphic marker locus, may or may not locate a single gene. A case might be made that the mode of inheritance of language impairment in this British family could, for instance, involve multiple genes. Other inherited disorders, such as breast cancer, are posited to have a number of plausible candidate genes that may be responsible for the disease (Hall et al., 1990). Researchers doing linkage studies in the area of inherited breast cancer have noted that "for those [families] in which inherited susceptibility for the disease does occur, different genes on different chromosomes could be responsible" (King, 1991, p. 123).

However, there is considerable evidence that the disorder in this family is the result of a single, autosomally dominant gene. Inherited susceptibility for a number of noncancerous disorders, such as retinoblastoma, has been linked to a particular single gene. Furthermore, it is this single gene that is altered in both inherited cases and in what are called *somatic* or *spontaneous* mutations. In the inheritance of the disorder in the particular family reported in this chapter, there is always a single affected parent, with no skipped generations, and the ratio of affected to unaffected members is 1:1. These factors are compatible with autosomal dominant single-gene modes of inheritance. However, this does not negate the possibility of more than one gene being affected, even if there is a pattern of autosomal dominant inheritance. Such genetic variation would be possible if linkage in one family is at one locus, and linkage in another family is at another locus. Research pertaining to the genetic basis of language impairment, then, needs to proceed to the stage of implementing linkage studies with several different families, for the likely possibility of inheritance by a single gene to be confirmed.

However, in order to ascertain genetic linkage, it is essential to define an adequate phenotype, the inheritance of which will be traced in families. "Real linkages can be missed and spurious linkages suggested either by defining the phenotype too broadly (so that persons without inherited susceptibility to disease are mistakenly categorized as affected) or simply by making errors in diagnosis" (Hall et al., 1990, p. 250). In the pursuit of establishing the genetic basis for language impairment, research will need to add the specification of a language-disordered phenotype to the already existing epidemiological ascertainment of family aggregations and to the case studies of large family aggregates. A phenotype is a description of a disorder that can eventually be matched to a genotype. To define such a phenotype, linguistically based accounts of the underlying grammar of SLI individuals are needed. The present omnibus tests and language analysis procedures used in communication disorders do not seem to target linguistic deficits thoroughly and specifically enough to serve this purpose. Multiple phenotypic measures may be needed, which may mean proceeding beyond the current clinical wisdom about what possible phenotypes might be or what the necessary cutoff points are for inclusion in a phenotype. Issues of some of what might be important to include in the specification of the phenotype for SLI emerge, when we consider the linguistic findings from the analyses of the language of the large family aggregate just described.

LINGUISTIC IMPAIRMENT IN THE LARGE FAMILY AGGREGATE

The linguistic data in the remainder of this chapter are taken from different aspects of the previously described family's language. The data include samples of spontaneous spoken and written language, as well as a series of tasks designed to tap various aspects of production and comprehension. The language data from affected members of the family come from individuals over 10 years of age; therefore, they can be considered linguistically mature. SLI has been documented to persist into adulthood (Tomblin, Freese, & Records, 1992). Understanding the final state of adult affected grammar is an important precondition to understanding the acquisition of language by SLI children. The possible grammars that can account for nonimpaired developing children's language are constrained by the general properties of language and by the specific grammatical properties of the particular language being acquired. However, these two constraints do not hold for affected language. Therefore, it is important to understand the final state grammar associated with language impairment, so that developing grammars of children affected by SLI can be related to the constraints of the potential final form.

The description of this family's language is based on linguistic principles articulated by Panini approximately 1,000 years ago (Gopnik, 1992). In brief, these principles include the following: explicit linguistic utterances are guided by internalized underlying rules, and the surface forms of the language do not constitute the language. It is the underlying grammar that needs to be characterized, and individual surface forms are less than representative of the underlying grammar. Furthermore, the grammar needs to be considered as a whole system. The following data, in fact, show that, although the surface forms produced by affected family members resemble surface forms produced by the nonaffected developing members, very different underlying processes seem to be at work in the grammar and in the way that language is learned. The language of this family is described in terms of three overriding categories: obligatory marking, obligatory consistency/agreement, and symbolic rules.

Obligatory Marking

Data from the affected family members show that they do not construct an obligatory category TENSE in the syntax and therefore do not obligatorily mark TENSE on the verb (Gopnik, in press). They do, however, encode a sense of *pastness* lexically by using phrases such as "and then." For instance, in spontaneous speech, the nonaffected family members all mark *past* correctly in a past context. The affected family members are quite different, producing verbs unmarked for past with error rates ranging from 14% to 70%. The most frequently occurring erroneous form was the stem. It could be argued that this stem form is a substitution of the present marking for the past marking because the present tense form resembles the stem for all persons in English, except for the third person singular. If this were true, the affected family members would be showing that they obligatorily mark TENSE, albeit the wrong tense on their verbs. However, in the 31 past tense contexts with the third person singular, the -s marked form occurred only three times. This indicates that it is the unmarked stem, not the present, that is used by the affected subjects.

The affected subjects also had trouble with a cloze procedure in which they had to change tense (Gopnik, in press). In this task, subjects were presented with a sentence in one tense and then offered the beginning of a sentence that required a tense change in the same verb for appropriate completion (e.g., Everyday the boy is happy. Yesterday he. . . .). There was a significant difference in the performance of the nonaffected and the affected subjects. The nonaffected subjects were right 92% of the time, while the affected subjects were correct only 38% of the time. Their errors and comments indicated that they had trouble understanding that they needed to manipulate tense. For instance, one family member gave the following response: "Everyday the boy is happy. Yesterday he *is unhappy.*"

On a rating task, the subjects were asked to rate certain sentences on a scale from one (unnatural sounding) to seven (natural sounding) (Gopnik, in press). For example, the following set of sentences would be given to a subject to rate:

> Bill was expecting his phone to ring at any moment.
> Still, when it rang he was surprised.
> Still, when it ringed, he was surprised.
> Still, when it ring he was surprised.

Similar sets using verbs with regular past tense endings were also administered. The results for this task concurred with the findings from the spontaneous speech. The affected subjects rated the stem form as somewhat acceptable, with a mean rating of 4.28. The nonaffected family members, however, found the stem form unacceptable, with a mean rating of 1.28. Again, it could be hypothesized that the affected members thought the stem form was the present tense and that they really knew that tense was obligatory. However, the majority of the items used the third person singular and would have required an -s ending to be interpreted as present tense. The remaining items, which did not require -s, were not rated as more acceptable. Therefore, it is not correct to assume that the affected subjects' performance reflected an error in agreement. Their judgments show that they found it acceptable to leave a verb unmarked for tense.

Obligatory Consistency/Agreement

The affected subjects showed particular difficulty in using tenses sequentially while making brief narrative descriptions of sequential pictures. No non-affected subjects changed tense while telling their stories, whereas all affected subjects violated local tense consistency constraints. This produced sentences such as, "The boy climbed and then the boy falls." Stem forms were frequently used, for example, "The boy climbed the tree and then the boy fall."

The affected subjects also differed significantly from the nonaffected subjects on the number of noun phrases they used when telling their narratives. For example, they used significantly fewer pronominal references than the nonaffected subjects did. This could be attributed to an inability to establish consistency or agreement between the pronoun and the preceding noun. This performance with anaphoric pronouns differed markedly from the affected members' ability to comprehend and use exophoric pronouns successfully. An alternative interpretation of the same performance is that the subjects did not establish pronominal reference because they were avoiding use of the pronominal structure. Such avoidance could be due to the fact that pronominal structure is more grammatically complex than the noun phrase.

Clahsen (1989) has described a theory for SLI based on German data that predict lack of agreement in certain parts of the grammar, for example, between the number and gender on nouns and their corresponding adjectives and articles in the noun phrase, between the noun and the verb, and with case markings. In English, agreement occurs in the noun phrase with regard to number, and in the verb phrase with regard to tense and noun–verb agreement. Preliminary investigation of agreement with the British subjects shows that the affected members have more difficulty with past tense agreement in their spontaneous speech than the nonaffected subjects do.

Findings about agreement in the noun phrase are also preliminary. There are sporadic examples of lack of agreement throughout the affected subjects' spontaneous speech (e.g., "a restaurants"). Also, in a task wherein the affected subjects were asked to correct items, some of them indicated that certain sentences, such as, "He had a pictures" were acceptable to them. Rice and Oetting (1993) have made a distinction between the performance of children with SLI in the noun phrase (*agr*) and agreement between the noun and the verb (*AGR*). In their study, children with SLI did have significantly more difficulty with noun–verb agreement than with agreement within the NP. Although no large-scale difficulties with NP agreement were found, some subtle differences were noted (cf. Rice & Oetting). Ongoing investigation into consistency and agreement across the grammar of the affected members of this family will be interesting to pursue.

Symbolic Rules

The data show that the affected subjects differ from their nonaffected peers on language tasks that involve the use of abstract procedural rules. Pinker (1991) has pointed out that there is a dual mechanism for learning to specify past tense. Past tense can be specified on regular verbs by the rule to add -*ed,* and on irregular verbs by learning a set of exceptions, which is accomplished by lexical memory and is affected by frequency of occurrence. It is assumed that, because the affected subjects do not have an obligatory category for tense in their grammar, they cannot construct a general symbolic rule based on tense. However, their differential learning of irregular past tense forms implies that they use a general associative memory system for learning.

Notebooks written by two of the family members with SLI demonstrate that they perform differently when using the regular and irregular past tense forms of verbs in their written narratives (Gopnik & Crago, 1991). The percentage of irregular verbs with the correct past form was far greater than the percentage of correct regular past forms. These affected subjects usually noted the irregular forms correctly on their first use of them. However, the regular past tense endings were learned only with repeated correction of the past tense for each specific verb, and rarely were they generalized to other verbs.

Similarly, the affected subjects could not use rule-governed behavior to mark singular and plural on nonsense words when they were shown pictures of imaginary animals (Gopnik & Crago, 1991).

UNDERLYING ASSUMPTIONS

The assumptions in the claim that a defective gene can cause language impairment require further investigation. They raise such questions as, is SLI with a genetic etiology different than SLI of an unknown etiology? Can language impairment be genetically based, even without a pattern of inheritance?

Group Comparisons

Certain group studies are necessary to begin to answer these questions. First, group comparisons of language impairment across family aggregations are needed. To determine the extent of interfamily variability, the language deficits suggested by Gopnik (in press) and Gopnik and Crago (1991) that occur in this British family must be compared in a systematic way with data from other families. Furthermore, a comparison of groups of SLI individuals with and without susceptibility for inheritance must be made. Such a comparison would provide information on whether different etiologies of SLI produce different forms of language impairment. Tallal, Townsend, Curtiss, and Wulfeck (1991) have compared individuals with SLI who have positive family histories to individuals with SLI who have negative family histories on a number of measures. Their results led these authors to conclude that "family history did not differentiate significantly between degree or pattern of language deficit" (p. 94). Tallal and her colleagues also concluded that the phenotypic profile for children with positive family histories was consistent with attentional and perceptual deficits. However, their conclusions were made without a thorough, linguistically based study of the subjects' language—in other words, without a carefully defined linguistic phenotype. Aggregation studies of the type that Tallal and her colleagues carried out are likely to produce different results than studies that employ a carefully defined phenotype for language.

Group comparisons based on a carefully and linguistically defined phenotype have some interesting possible implications. For instance, if the language impairment found in individuals with positive family histories is, in fact, the same as that found in individuals with negative family histories, this could indicate that differing etiologies do not lead to differing forms of language impairment. Such a finding would imply that the language system has vulnerable aspects that can break down in similar ways due to a variety of causes. However, such similarities would not necessarily mean that SLI is not genetically caused. It could mean that there is no foolproof way to distinguish between genetic and inherited patterns of language impairment. In other words, the phenotypes caused by spontaneous somatic mutations and inheritance would not be different. In the breast cancer example cited earlier, women who are susceptible to inheriting this disease do not have a different form of breast cancer than women with no genetic susceptibility. They do, however, develop it at a characteristically earlier age. A problem in differentiation also occurs at the genetic level because alterations in genes caused by spontaneous mutation and inheritability can be, in some ways, indistinguishable (King, 1991). In both cases, the genetic alteration occurs at the level of the DNA. However, if the criterion of occurrence in families is applied, then spontaneous mutation and inheritance are, a priori, distinguishable. Furthermore, it is assumed that genetic alterations can cause changes in the neural substrate, possibly of the kind that Plante (1991) and Plante et al. (1991) documented. Again, inherited changes at the neurological level might not be distinguishable from changes at that level that might occur from spontaneous genetic mutation.

It is also interesting to speculate on the possible meaning of group comparisons that would show differences in the language of individuals with positive and negative family histories. Possibly, spontaneous genetic mutations could appear in families with a negative history, and these could result in a different performance from that of individuals with inherited genes, or differences between the groups could mean that some individuals with SLI do not have a genetic basis for their language impairment. In this case, different etiologies for SLI could be seen to cause different forms of language impairment or different degrees of severity.

It is also plausible to assume that, rather than a "gene for grammar," as certain media reported, there might be genetic alterations to an ability or a variety of abilities that include or underlie grammatical abilities. At present, the claim is that there is an impaired gene that affects grammar (Gopnik, 1992). What is not known, until further research is undertaken, is how such a gene affects grammar. The presence of such an impaired gene is not implausible, and, indeed, certain researchers have claimed that individuals affected by language impairment have a number of cognitive deficits (Johnston, 1993). Future research must address whether such cognitive deficits are causal or concomitant with language impairment and how, if at all, they are related to the genetic basis for language impairment. Claiming that language is impaired and that there is an impaired gene is not equivalent to describing the specifics of how these two factors fit together. There are a few different possible fits. It may be that the impaired gene causes some form of cognitive deficit that is at the base of a language deficit, or it may be that it causes only a language deficit. It also remains uncertain whether the impaired gene(s) causes specific language impairment alone, rather than a set of associated disabilities.

Individual Variation

Finally, there is another question. What is the meaning of the individual variation that exists in the familial aggregations of language impairment? Certainly, in the British family studied, individual members manifested a range of language behaviors (Gopnik & Crago, 1991). Work is presently under way on how to represent such individual variations in a meaningful way. In the meantime, a number of possible interpretations might explain such variation on both a genetic and a linguistic level. On the genetic level, the variation might reflect how large the insertion of DNA is in the gene. Studies of the inheritance of myotonic dystrophy and the Fragile X syndrome show increasing severity over generations, reflecting the increasing size of the insertion over generations (Fu et al., 1992). New genetic evidence suggests that it may even be the case that individual differences across families might result from whether the gene is expressed through the mother or the father (Brzustowicz, 1991; Tomblin, 1991).

On the linguistic level, individual variation might also reflect different degrees of compensation by various family members. This, in turn, might reflect different amounts or types of intervention or different degrees of compensating cognitive strategies and/or abilities. For instance, the higher intelligence levels of certain affected individuals may help them to develop more effective communication strategies. Similarly, different individual memory capacities probably interact with various individuals' language impairment to create greater and lesser degrees of compensation. If, for example, the past tense form of irregular verbs relies on an associative memory strategy for learning, then, greater memory capacity may well result in better language attainment.

IMPLICATIONS FOR CLINICAL LANGUAGE SAMPLING

Surface Forms

Analysis of the language data of the British family has implications for a number of assumptions and procedures used in clinical investigations of language impairment. Clinical language sampling procedures generally rely on counts of surface forms (Crystal, Fletcher, & Garman, 1989; Fletcher, 1991; Lee & Canter, 1971; Miller, 1981, 1991; Saffran, Berndt, & Schwartz, 1989; Scarborough, 1990) without accounting for the underlying grammar. The net effect of this can be camouflaging of the underlying grammar. Verb stems, for instance, are not identified in a number of clinical analysis procedures. When they are, their relationship to the use of symbolic rules for past tense or for obligatory marking is not elaborated.

Surface forms for the present tense produced by affected members of this family often resemble the surface forms produced by the nonaffected family members. Such forms would be counted as correct in clinical language analysis systems. The surface forms for the past tense in the affected family members, when they were marked for past, also did not differ from the surface forms produced by the nonaffected subjects. However, the surface form used for the past was not always marked for tense. For instance, the subjects produced the following types of forms:

1. I walk. (for a present tense situation)
2. He walk. (for a present tense situation)
3. He walk. (for a past tense situation)

Clinical analysis systems would count the unmarked forms in numbers 2 and 3 as errors and number 1 would be seen as correct. In fact, we have no way of knowing whether tense is marked on number 1. A problem in the obligatory marking of tense implies that there is a problem in both present and past tense. So, while the affected members do show evidence of a past tense form, they do not have a rule that allows them to mark tense obligatorily. This distinction between different surface forms is not reflected in the present scoring of surface forms on clinical systems of language analysis.

Error Analysis

Full investigation of language requires not only the calculation of the percentages correct and incorrect, but also an analysis of the errors. To define patterns of language behavior, it is important to investigate the nature of the errors, by differentiating them from one another.

For instance, the nature of the error in past tense in the following examples needs to be differentiated:

1. flied/flew
2. fly/flew
3. The girl went to the doctor because she is ill.

Information on whether the erroneous form is a stem (*fly*), or an incorrectly inflected past (*flied*), or lack of consistency across the sentence clarifies the nature of the deficit.

Analysis Across the Grammar

The relationship of forms across the grammar also reveals underlying mechanisms. For example, Pinker's (1991) dual mechanism hypothesis predicts that the learning of past tense rules for regular verbs contrasts with the learning of the past tense forms for irregular verbs in important ways. It is important, then, to relate these two components to each other. Clahsen's (1989) agreement hypothesis relates errors in article agreement, plurals, third person singular, and copula to each other because they all indicate problems with agreement. Rice and Oetting (1993) would distinguish agreement in the noun phrase, such as article agreement, from agreement in the verb phrases, such as third person singular. In clinical analysis systems, the parts of the grammar seem to be like separate glasses which, for full proficiency, need to be filled up one at a time. Instead, it might be hypothesized that they are a system of glasses connected at the base by tubes. In such systems, liquid filling one glass will have an impact on the other parts of the system.

Partial Mastery

Our interpretation of this family's language impairment raises questions concerning clinical notions about partial mastery. Their variable use of certain morphological inflections has been considered to be a part of the evidence for a lack of rule-governed behavior in language. This interpretation seems to contrast with Miller's (1981) interpretation of variability:.

> It would not be satisfactory to accept the criterion of 90% and say that Jay does not "have," for example, a contractible copula. He clearly *has* it, since he uses it about 50% of the time, and in writing a grammar we must assume that it is generated in instances by a rule. We want the grammar to provide a mechanism for producing variable forms, although we may set aside for the moment why they are used variably. (p. 87)

Data from this family indicate that, when a person uses a morpheme 50% of the time, it may not be warranted to assume that this person "has" that grammatical form. It does, however, indicate that the delineation of a rule for the use of that form is either incomplete or incorrect. In fact, taken with other evidence, a 50%, or even a 90%, "mastery" score might constitute proof that Jay did not have a completely delineated rule for generating his grammar.

Variable production of grammatical forms, then, is an important feature of children's impaired language that must be accounted for. Partial mastery has been more typically viewed as an indicator of incomplete development, as though the capacity to produce a grammatical form was, to repeat the previous metaphor, like a partially filled glass. Maturation or intervention has been expected to fill the glass. Instead, partial mastery or variable use of a form, such as the past tense *-ed* morpheme, could indicate incomplete delineation of rule-governed behavior, wherein something has not clicked in the affected person's mind from the beginning, but wherein certain surface forms are present because compensatory strategies, such as lexical associative learning, have provided access to them in the absence of a rule-governed strategy.

Goals of Assessment and Intervention

If the goals of assessment are to identify affected individuals or to match populations on the surface characteristics of their grammar, then many of our clinical tools suffice. If, however, a clinical analysis of a child's language is intended to provide an account of the underlying grammar or an account of why a child's language is deficient, then clinical analyses procedures must be revised. The underlying patterns that will predict hierarchical and interactional relationships in principled ways must be explored so that language and its learning can be appropriately characterized. Without this level of characterization, certain intervention efforts may be misguided. For instance, the concept of a dual mechanism for language learning applied to language impairment would imply that lexical learning strategies for verbal morphemes are a more profitable avenue for intervention than rule-based intervention. The nature of compensatory strategies used by children with SLI in their language acquisition must be studied. Detailed investigation of the language of family aggregations should lead to distinctions between the immutable aspects of language and the mutable ones, so that the mutable aspects can become the focus of intervention.

CONCLUSIONS

Empirical evidence from the study of a large family aggregate with SLI has led to claims about the genetic basis of language, the representation of language in the brain, the nature of its acquisition, and the innate properties of language. More genetic and linguistic evidence is necessary to substantiate these claims and to bring a more complete understanding of the properties of genetically impaired and nonimpaired language.

REFERENCES

Bishop, D.V.M. (1992). The biological basis of specific language impairment. In P. Fletcher & D. Hall (Eds.), *Specific language disorders in children: Correlates, characteristics, and outcomes* (pp. 2–17). San Diego, CA: Singular Publishing Group.

Bombeck, E. (1992). *Lousy grammar? It must be lousy genes.* Kansas City: Universal Press Syndicate.

Borges-Osorio, M.R.L., & Salzano, F.M. (1985). Language disabilities in three twin pairs and their relatives. *Acta Geneticae Medicae Gemellologiae, 34,* 95–100.

Brzustowicz, L.M. (1991, November). *The revolution in human genetics.* Paper presented at the American Speech-Language-Hearing Association on Genetics: Progress and promise for communication sciences and disorders, Atlanta, GA.

Clahsen, H. (1989). The grammatical characterization of developmental dysphasia. *Linguistics, 27,* 897–920.

Crystal, D., Fletcher, P., & Garman, M. (1989). *Grammatical analysis of language disability.* London, UK: Whurr.

Fitzgerald, K. (1992). Talking genes. *The Sciences, 32*(3), 7–8.

Fletcher, P. (1991). Evidence from syntax for language impairment. In J.F. Miller (Ed.), *Research on child language disorders* (pp. 169–188). Austin, TX: PRO-ED.

Fu, Y.-H., Pizzuti, A., Fenwick, R.G. Jr., King, J., Rajnarayan, S., Dunne, P.W., Dubei, J., Nasser, G.A., Ashizawa, T., de Jong, P., Wieringa, B., Korneluk, R., Perryman, M.B., Epstein, H.F., & Caskey, C.T. (1992). An unstable triplet repeat in a gene related to myotonic muscular dystrophy. *Science, 255,* 1256–1258.

Gopnik, M. (1992, February). *Linguistic properties of genetic language impairment.* Paper presented at the American Association for the Advancement of Science Conference, Chicago, IL.

Gopnik, M. (in press). Impairments of syntactic tense in a familial language disorder. *Journal of Neurolinguistics.*

Gopnik, M., & Crago, M.B. (1991). Familial aggregation of a developmental language disorder. *Cognition, 39,* 1–50.

Gopnik, M., & Crago, M. (in press). Genetic dysphasia: Issues and explanations. *McGill Working Papers in Linguistics.*

Hall, J., Lee, M.K., Newman, B., Morrow, J.E., Anderson, L.A., Huey, B., & King, M.-C. (1990). Linkage to early onset familial breast cancer to chromosome 17q21. *Science, 250,* 1684–1689.

Hurst, J.A., Baraitser, M., Auger, E., Graham, F., & Norell, S. (1990). An extended family with a dominantly inherited speech disorder. *Neurology, 32,* 347–355.

Johnston, J.R. (1993). *Specific language impairment, cognition, and the biological basis of language.* Paper presented at the Sixth Vancouver Conference on Cognitive Sciences, The Biological Basis of Language, Vancouver, BC, Canada.

King, M.-C. (1991). Localization of the early-onset breast cancer gene. *Hospital Practice, 26,* 121–126.

Lee, L., & Canter, S. (1971). Developmental sentence scoring: A procedure for estimating syntactic development in children's spontaneous speech. *Journal of Speech and Hearing Disorders, 36,* 315–340.

Lewis, B., & Thompson, L. (1992). A study of developmental speech and language disorders in twins, *Journal of Speech and Hearing Research, 35,* 1086–1094.

Miller, J.F. (1981). *Assessing language production in children.* Baltimore: University Park Press.

Miller, J.F. (1991). Quantifying productive language disorders. In J.F. Miller (Ed.), *Research on child language disorders* (pp. 211–220). Austin, TX: PRO-ED.

Pembrey, M. (1992). Genetics and language disorders. In P. Fletcher & D. Hall (Eds.), *Specific language disorders in children: Correlates, characteristics, and outcomes* (pp. 51–62). San Diego: Singular Publishing Group.

Pinker, S. (1991). Rules of language. *Science, 253,* 530–535.

Plante, E. (1991). MRI findings in boys with specific language impairment. *Brain and Language, 41*(1), 67–80.

Plante, E., Swisher, L., Vance, R., & Rapcsak, S. (1991). MRI findings in parents and siblings of specifically language-impaired boys. *Brain and Language, 41*(1), 52–66.

Rice, M.L., & Oetting, J.B. (1993). Morphological deficits of children with SLI: Evaluation of number marking and agreement. *Journal of Speech and Hearing Research, 36*, 1249–1257.

Saffran, E.M., Berndt, R.S., & Schwartz, M. (1989). The quantitative analysis of agrammatic productions: Procedure and data. *Brain and Language, 37*, 440–479.

Samples, J.M., & Lane, V.W. (1985). Genetic possibilities in six siblings with specific language learning disorders. *Asha, 27*, 27–32.

Scarborough, H. (1990). Index of productive syntax. *Applied Psycholinguistics, 11*(1), 1–22.

Tallal, P., Ross, R., & Curtiss, S. (1989). Familial aggregation in specific language impairment. *Journal of Speech and Hearing Disorders, 54*, 167–173.

Tallal, P., Townsend, J., Curtiss, S., & Wulfeck, B. (1991). Phenotypic profiles of language-impaired children based on genetic/family history. *Brain and Language, 41*, 81–95.

Tomblin, J.B. (1989). Familial concentration of developmental language impairment. *Journal of Speech and Hearing Disorders, 54*, 287–295.

Tomblin, B. (1991, November). *Inquiries into the genetics of specific language impairment.* Paper presented at the Annual Convention of the American Speech-Language-Hearing Association, Atlanta, GA.

Tomblin, J.B., Freese, P.R., & Records, N.L. (1992). Diagnosing specific language impairment in adults for the purpose of pedigree analysis. *Journal of Speech and Hearing Research, 35*, 832–843.

4

Grammatical Challenges for Children with Specific Language Impairments

Ruth V. Watkins

A NUMBER OF RECENT STUDIES have identified particular linguistic construc-
tions that prove challenging for children with specific language impairments.
For example, syntactic features such as grammatical morphemes have consistently been identified as troublesome for language-impaired children (Lahey,
Liebergott, Chesnick, Menyuk, & Adams, 1992; Leonard, 1989; Leonard,
Bortolini, Caselli, McGregor, & Sabbadini, 1992; Rice & Oetting, 1991;
Watkins & Rice, 1991). Much of this work has served as a foundation for
current accounts of specific language impairment; several recent theories of
language impairment are built around consistently documented grammatical
difficulties evidenced by this population (Clahsen, 1989, 1991; Gopnik &
Crago, 1991; Leonard et al., 1992).

Two divergent theories have focused specifically on accounting for the
particular problem-space constituted by morphology. In one position, Gopnik
and Crago (1991) posited that children with language impairments are missing
many features of the grammatical system, such as number, tense, and aspect.
This position was developed primarily through detailed study of a single
three-generation family, containing 16 affected (SLI) and 14 nonaffected
members. A series of linguistic probes revealed that family members with SLI
demonstrated particular difficulty in marking number, tense, and aspect features of the grammar. Based on these data, the missing features hypothesis
predicts that children with SLI will fail to master fully a wide range of basic
grammatical contrasts marking these grammatical features; some random correct application or partial mastery is thought to be possible by way of rote
learning of specific words.

In a competing account of SLI children's grammatical deficits, Leonard
and his colleagues (Leonard, 1989, chap. 6, this volume) propose that the
ability to perceive, process, and develop generalized linguistic rules about
brief, unstressed aspects of the grammatical system is disrupted in children

with SLI. This position is founded on the analysis of English morphological acquisition patterns, as well as study of morpheme acquisition in other languages. Through cross-linguistic study of SLI children's mastery of morphological forms, Leonard has identified inflectional morphemes that prove particularly difficult; one common thread among these constructions, according to this account, is their low phonetic substance (i.e., brief duration and limited stress, cf. Leonard et al., 1992). Although the surface hypothesis emphasizes the challenge of brief, unstressed aspects of the grammar, the account is not completely restricted to the perceptual level. For example, Leonard predicts that the final -s in a plural grammatical context would be easier for children with SLI than the final -s in a third person verb grammatical context, because the plural marker has a relatively straightforward semantic correlate. However, as yet, the specific contribution of semantic and or syntactic factors has not been clearly delineated by the surface account.

One challenge to evaluating these two accounts is that each is supported by certain aspects of available data on the grammatical deficits of children with SLI. In turn, evidence exists that is inconsistent with both the missing features and the surface accounts. In order to evaluate these positions fully, and to construct more complete accounts, the performance of children with SLI on a wider range of linguistic skills must be appraised. To this end, findings from three studies of the semantic–syntactic abilities of children with SLI are reviewed in this chapter. Associations between these findings and the two current accounts of SLI are then considered; the central purpose of this discussion is to reflect on how aspects of the linguistic system that are particularly problematic for children with SLI relate to current accounts of the disorder. Finally, implications of these grammatical limitations for clinical practice are highlighted.

RESEARCH ON GRAMMATICAL CHALLENGES

Acquisition of Particles and Prepositions

The first grammatical challenge involves verb particles and prepositions. This study investigated the acquisition of verb particle and prepositional phrase structures in children with language impairment and in nonaffected children (Watkins & Rice, 1991). A verb particle construction involves a multiword grammatical unit that functions as a verb. For example, in the sentence *kick over the fence,* the verb *kick* and the particle *over* function together as a grammatical unit. The verb particle can also be defined in contrast to the preposition structure. Verb particles may either precede or follow full lexical noun phrases (e.g., *put on the hat, put the hat on*); however, they must follow a pronominal noun phrase (e.g., *put it on* vs. **put on it*). In contrast, prepositions always precede their noun objects, whether full or pronominal (e.g., *sit* *on the chair, sit on it*) (Bolinger, 1971; Dixon, 1982; Fraser, 1976; Goodluck, 1986; Quirk, Greenbaum, Leech, & Svartvik, 1985).

The primary motivation for examining verb particle and preposition constructions is that they allow evaluation of Leonard's (1989) surface hypothesis. Particles and prepositions involve identical surface forms of brief duration and relatively limited stress that contrast in underlying structural representations. Whereas prepositions conform to consistent word order, particles permit varied word order. Furthermore, particles require a shift in the pronominal that prepositions do not. The surface account predicts that both forms should pose difficulty for children with SLI; if differential difficulty were identified, the influence of more general semantic and syntactic factors may be involved.

A total of 42 preschool-age children participated in this study, 14 children with specific language impairments, 14 chronological age–matched children, and 14 language-matched children. The children with SLI ranged in age from 4;5 to 5;7, and met relatively standard criteria for SLI; that is, they had been diagnosed as having a language impairment by a certified speech-language pathologist, and had normal intellectual skills and hearing abilities. In addition, they displayed the following linguistic deficits: 1) a score one or more standard deviations below the mean on the Peabody Picture Vocabulary Test–Revised (Dunn & Dunn, 1981); 2) mean length of utterance (MLU) one or more standard deviations below the mean; and 3) lack of mastery of three or more grammatical morphemes. The age- and language-matched children demonstrated normal intelligence, hearing, and social-emotional development, as well as PPVT–R standard scores and MLU within or above the normal range.

A videotaped task was developed to elicit six verb particle and preposition words (*over, in, on, off, up,* and *down*) in both full noun phrase and pronominal noun phrase contexts. The same words were evaluated in both particle and preposition linguistic contexts. The target measure was the children's production of particles and prepositions.

The basic design used in this study was a four-way mixed analysis of variance (ANOVA), with group as a between-subjects factor (language-impaired, age-matched, language-matched), and grammatical context (particle, preposition), linguistic context (full noun phrase, pronominal noun phrase), and word (*in, on, off, over, up, down*) as within-subjects factors. The primary result of the study was a significant three-way interaction of group $\times$ grammatical context $\times$ linguistic context ($F(2,39) = 3.48$, $p < .01$). This interaction is displayed in Figure 1. Inspection of the figure suggests that the interaction occurred in the preposition context; this was confirmed by follow-up tests.

In the particle grammatical context, the age-matched group performed significantly better than the language-matched group and the language-matched group performed significantly more accurately than the language-

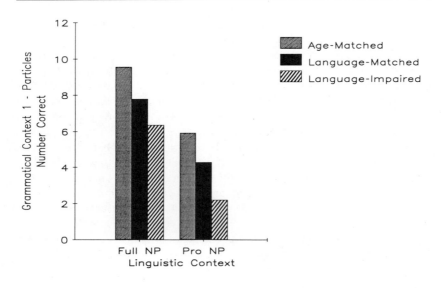

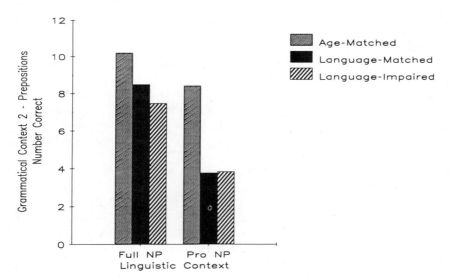

Figure 1. Verb particle and preposition acquisition; group × grammatical context × linguistic context inter-action.

impaired group. In the preposition grammatical context, however, the age-matched group performed significantly better than the language-impaired group on full noun phrase items, while the language-impaired group and the language-matched groups did not differ in performance. The same pattern occurred for the pronominal noun phrase items within the preposition grammatical context; the age-matched group differed from both the language-matched and the language-impaired groups, while the performance of the language-impaired group and the language-matched group was equivalent.

In summary, the primary finding of this study was that verb particles constituted a particularly challenging grammatical task for children with language impairment. In contrast, such children performed like their younger, typically developing counterparts on preposition items, items that were identical surface forms/words.

The specific pattern of difficulty with particle acquisition evidenced by the children with language impairment is predicted by Leonard's (1989) surface account. However, the finding that the same surface forms, when used as prepositions, were less problematic, is not well captured by the surface hypothesis. Instead, this pattern of difficulty suggests that more generalized semantic and syntactic factors have greater influence than is acknowledged or clearly predicted by the surface account. In terms of the missing features account, verb particles do not correspond to as yet identified features of grammatical difficulty in a straightforward manner.

Candidate explanations for the specific difficulty evidenced by the SLI subjects with particles include the fact that particles are syntactically and semantically more complex than prepositions. For example, particles depend on the verb stem, combining with it to form a multiword verb unit; prepositions function independently of the verb. Difficulties with particle forms could be tied to more general and pervasive difficulties with verb acquisition and use. Because particle constructions involve multiword verb plus particle combinations, a limited verb lexicon may impede particle use and accuracy.

Verb Acquisition and Use

The second grammatical challenge involves verb use by children with SLI. Although delayed lexical acquisition in children with language impairment has been relatively well documented in recent literature (Leonard, 1988; Rice, 1991; Rice, Buhr, & Nemeth, 1990), the majority of this work has focused on nouns. To date, limited research has addressed acquisition of verbs in children with language impairment. One study available in this area, conducted by Fletcher and Peters (1984), observed that children with language impairment used a more restricted set of verbs than their age-matched counterparts; a younger language-matched comparison group was not included in the Fletcher and Peters study. In a related investigation, Rice and Bode (1993) examined the spontaneous verb usage of three preschool-age children with specific language impairments. Analysis of transcript data revealed that the children used a relatively restricted set of verbs to fulfill a majority of verb functions. Rice and Bode termed these high-frequency forms general all-purpose (GAP) verbs, and documented that, although the youngsters with SLI used this set heavily, they generally did so in a grammatically correct manner (i.e., appropriate argument structures were generally associated with GAP verbs). Although this study provides key information about the verb profiles of three children with SLI through transcript data, it does not include comparison with nonaffected children.

In the study to be discussed, then, Watkins, Rice, and Moltz (1993) aimed to contrast the diversity and type of verb forms used by children with language impairment with those of two nonaffected comparison groups, one matched to the children with language impairment on the basis of age, and the other on the basis of language ability. In addition to the hint provided by difficulty with particles, this interest in verb learning is triggered by the notion that verb properties influence and direct many other aspects of grammar (Gleitman, 1989; Pinker, 1989). Basic descriptions of verb form use of children with language impairment have the potential to provide an insight into the nature and character of early language delay, and can suggest directions for additional work in this area.

Forty-two preschool-age children participated in this study, 14 children with specific language impairment, 14 language-matched children, and 14 age-matched children. The subject selection criteria implemented in this study parallel those used in the particle–preposition study discussed above. The subjects with language impairment were 59.5 months of age, with an average MLU of 3.29. The language-matched subjects were 38.1 months of age, with a mean MLU of 3.35. The age-matched subjects averaged 60.9 months of age.

A 100-utterance sample of each subject's productive language, collected with a standard toy kit, was analyzed for: 1) main verb type-token ratio (TTR), a measure of main verb diversity; and 2) frequently used main verb forms (verb types occurring with greater than average frequency, following a procedure developed by Rice & Bode, 1993). A list of high-frequency verbs was then made for each subject group, and the percentage of verb types and verb tokens accounted for by these high-frequency forms was calculated.

First, in terms of verb TTR, a one-way ANOVA was used to compare the main verb type-token ratios of the three subject groups. This analysis revealed a significant group effect (F [2,19] = 3.50, $p < .05$). The mean verb TTR for the language-impaired group was 0.42; for the language-matched group, 0.50; and for the age-matched group, 0.48. Follow-up analyses revealed significant differences between the language-impaired and language-matched groups, and between the language-impaired and age-matched groups. Differences between the language-matched and age-matched groups were not significant.

In addition, analysis of overall TTR revealed nonsignificant differences between subject groups ($M = 0.45$).

Second, a number of high-frequency verbs were identified for each subject group. There were 15 high-frequency forms for the language-impaired group, 19 for the language-matched group, and 22 for the age-matched group. Eleven of the high-frequency verbs were common across all three subject groups—do, go, get, got, put, want, know, open, play, see, and look. These high-frequency verbs constituted approximately 28%–29% of the subjects' verb types, and roughly 58%–60% of the subjects' verb tokens, a finding comparable across subject groups. However, it is useful to recall that the SLI subjects used 15 high-frequency verb forms, the language-matched subjects 19, and the age-matched subjects 22; yet, these high-frequency forms comprised equivalent percentages of the verb types and tokens used by all the subject groups.

Analysis of main verb TTRs revealed that the subjects with language impairment relied on a more limited set of verb forms than did their language- and age-matched peers. This finding is striking because the 5-year-old children with language impairment demonstrated less verb diversity than did the 3-year-old nonaffected children at the same language level, in addition to the deficit expected when compared to age-matched peers.

These results provide basic descriptive information on verb use in children with specific language impairments, relative to their peers without language impairments. The finding of a strong degree of overlap in high-frequency forms is not particularly surprising, when factors such as verb frequency in adult language and the general utility of the high-occurrence forms are considered. More surprising, however, is the evidence of limited main verb diversity found relative to age- and language-matched peers.

With respect to the two theoretical accounts of SLI, the limited verb diversity evidenced by the children with language impairment is not predicted clearly by either surface or missing features accounts. Although acquisition of verb forms is, at a basic level, a lexical challenge, limitations in the verb system have significant potential for relating to or triggering grammatical problems. For example, a limited verb lexicon may be linked to the difficulty evidenced in children with SLI in using verb particle constructions. Furthermore, limitations in the verb lexicon have the potential to delay morphological acquisition. Pinker's (1984, 1989) learnability model of grammatical acquisition suggests that children develop morphologic inflections by first building word-specific paradigms, wherein each lexical item and each inflected word constitute separate lexical entries. At some point, however, when a critical number of lexical entries have been made, children generate productive rules for inflection use. Thus, a limited verb system could slow the process of generating generalized paradigms for inflection use.

Moreover, restrictions in verb diversity would seem to conflict directly with a suggestion raised in Gopnik and Crago's (1991) missing feature perspective on SLI. They suggested that correct use of specific missing features (e.g., number or tense markers) is accounted for by rote learning of particular lexical forms, rather than generalized application of a grammatical rule. Given the limitations in verb system diversity documented here and word acquisition difficulties noted in other studies, it seems problematic to credit children with language impairment with robust lexical learning strategies as the vehicle for explaining occasional or emergent use of verb inflections.

Acquisition of One Derivational Morpheme

The third grammatical challenge deals with derivational morphology. As mentioned previously, morphology is one aspect of the grammar that has been documented to be problematic for children with a language impairment (cf. Johnston & Schery, 1976; Khan & James, 1983; Lahey et al., 1992; Leonard et al., 1992; Steckol & Leonard, 1979). Study in this area has frequently examined acquisition of Brown's 14 grammatical morphemes in SLI children, but it has not yet included assessment of derivational morphology. Derivational morphemes afford an additional avenue through which the grammatical skills of children with a language impairment can be assessed, chiefly because derivational forms share a number of features of grammatical morphology. For example, they are relatively brief, unstressed aspects of the grammar; thus, according to the surface account, they may challenge children with SLI. In addition, productive use of derivational forms requires application of abstract rules. Given the underlying deficit in the grammars of children with SLI proposed by the missing features account, derivational morphemes would also be predicted to be troublesome for children with SLI. For these reasons, derivational morphemes offer the possibility of aiding in the evaluation of current accounts of SLI.

The specific aims of this study were to assess the ability of children with SLI to use one derivational form, -er, relative to their age- and language-matched peers, and to contrast patterns of -er use with one inflectional morpheme, third person -s (Watkins, Buhr, & Davis, submitted). A videotape task was used to create a context in which 12 monosyllabic verbs (not derived from nouns and present in the speech of 3-year-olds, cf. Clark & Hecht, 1982) were elicited as agent or instrument nouns, or as their verb base. For example, the verb *cut* was used to elicit the -er derivational morpheme and the -s third person verb inflection with such prompts as, "This boy cuts things. A boy who cuts things is a _____" and, "This is a cutter. What does a cutter do?"

Forty children from four subject groups participated in the study. The three groups forming the primary analysis were: 1) 10 5-year-old children with specific language impairments, using criteria discussed previously; 2) 10 5-year-old children with normal language skills, matched to the subjects with a language impairment on the basis of age; and 3) 10 3-year-old children with normal language skills, matched to the language-impaired group on the basis of MLU. An additional group of 10 7-year-old children with language impairments participated in the study in order to provide information on morphological abilities in older SLI subjects.

The first question of this study was whether group differences would be identified in the use of the derivational morpheme -er in agent and instrument contexts. This analysis was conducted using a two-way mixed analysis of variance (ANOVA), with group as a between-subjects factor and semantic role (agent or instrument) as a within-subjects factor. Results revealed a significant interaction of group and semantic role (F [3,36] = 6.25, $p < .05$). Figure 2 illustrates this interaction. Comparison of performance on agent versus instrument items for each subject group revealed a significant difference for the 5-year-old subjects with language impairment only. Furthermore, follow-up analyses indicated that on agent items, the 5-year-old group with language impairment performed more poorly than their age-mates, but equivalent to their language-matched counterparts. In contrast, on instrument items, the 5-year-old language-impaired group performed more poorly than both their age- and language-matched peers. Finally, both the 5-year-old nonaffected

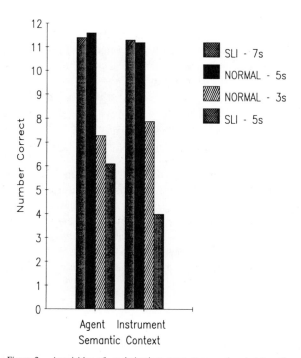

Figure 2. Acquisition of -er derivation; group × semantic role interaction.

subjects and the 7-year-old subjects with language impairment demonstrated mastery level performance (90% accuracy or greater) on both agent and instrument -er items.

The second question of this study was to assess the subjects' ability to use the third person -s verb inflection. A one-way ANOVA revealed a significant main effect for group (F [3,36] = 7.4, $p < .05$). Follow-up analyses showed a significant difference between the 5-year-old subjects with language impairment and their age- and language-matched peers. The 7-year-old subjects with SLI did not differ from the 3- and the 5-year-old children with typical language skills.

Three key aspects of these findings are of particular interest. First, the discrepancy noted between the 5-year-olds with SLI agent and instrument uses of the -er form for SLI suggests that surface attributes are only one contributing factor to acquisition; semantic factors also are likely to be influential. Second, the mastery level performance of 7-year-old subjects with SLI on agent and instrument -er items indicates that formation of general and productive grammatical rules in this population is not blocked, and full attainment of syntactic contrasts can occur. Third, divergent patterns of acquisition for the -er and third person -s morpheme suggest that aspects of the -s inflection render it particularly difficult for children with specific impairments. Possible explanations for this difficulty include some combination of very brief duration, semantic–syntactic complexity, and involvement of the verb system.

Relative to the current theoretical accounts of SLI, the difficulty evidenced by the 5-year-old subjects with SLI with instrument -er items is predicted by both surface and missing features accounts. In contrast, the discrepancy between the agent and instrument uses of -er in 5-year-old children with SLI is not clearly anticipated by either hypothesis. The surface account might attribute the divergence in performance to semantic distinctions between agent and instrument forms, but the account does not as yet clearly anticipate such a distinction.

Moreover, the mastery level use of -er evidenced by the 7-year-old children with SLI is problematic for the missing features perspective. If the formation of an abstract underlying rule for the -er derivation were missing, the mastery level of attainment evidenced by the 7-year-olds with SLI would be implausible or even impossible. The surface account, however, is less clear in predicting eventual levels of mastery, and might attribute the acquisition of -er in 7-year-olds with SLI to its duration and syllabic nature.

IMPLICATIONS FOR CURRENT ACCOUNTS OF SLI

In summary, findings from these three investigations reveal that the two current accounts of SLI, the missing features and surface hypotheses, are inadequate to account for the full range of observed empirical evidence on the grammatical challenges displayed by children with SLI. Although available theoretical positions accurately account for some aspects of the data, certain patterns of strength and vulnerability in the grammatical acquisition of children with SLI are not clearly linked to current theories. This is not to deny that there is considerable evidence consistent with both missing features and surface accounts. Rather, the intent is to suggest areas for expanding current accounts to encompass the broad range of challenges associated with specific language impairment.

In light of the range of difficulties identified here, the aspects of the language system likely to be influenced by these documented challenges, and existing knowledge of the broad scope of problems children with SLI have in diverse areas of language acquisition (e.g., lexicon, phonology, social aspects), the question of where these difficulties converge is likely to continue to be perplexing. The multifaceted problem of specific language impairment demands use of converging research methods and multidimensional approaches to theory building.

Converging Research Methods

A key avenue for extending our knowledge of SLI will be to pursue complementary sources of evidence about the disorder. Although available methodologies seem to be stretched to their limits in terms of what they can reveal about the nature and character of language impairment, varied research methods (i.e., different from the experimental, cross-sectional type used in the studies reported here) offer the potential to yield valuable insights. For example, Brown's (1973) longitudinal documentation of Adam, Eve, and Sarah's process of language development from single words through grammar has been and continues to be one of the single most informative sources of information in the field. As yet, a parallel study of similar scope of children with specific language impairment has not been conducted. Admittedly, the heterogeneity in children with specific language impairment could make subject selection challenging, and would require tracking the developmental patterns of a number of children. However, potential rewards in the form of information about the linguistic phenotype of specific language impairment, including developmental change and patterns of acquisition, are considerable.

Theory Building

Ultimately, the development of complete accounts of specific language impairment in children depends upon the integration of detailed information from a number of areas, including: 1) specification of the *linguistic characteristics* of specific language impairment; that is, identifying the full range of aspects of the language system that are impaired, and delineating which of those aspects are associated with an inherited pattern of disorder (i.e., linguistic phenotype); 2) documentation of *developmental changes* in the linguistic character of SLI; and 3) convergence of evidence from *cross-linguistic studies* of SLI. One clear aspect of available findings is that there may be multiple sources of vulnerability for the acquisition of various grammatical skills. As research and theoretical pursuits advance on varied aspects of the problem, our understanding of the nature of the disorder will advance similarly.

THE CLINICAL CHALLENGE

As noted throughout this chapter, children with specific language impairments demonstrate particular difficulty with numerous aspects of the grammatical system. The work reported here, as well as many other investigations, suggests that key areas of difficulty center on the morphological and verb systems. An important question to be addressed, then, involves both if and how these areas of difficulty can be related to clinical practice. Moreover, it should be noted that adopting either of the two current accounts of SLI—the missing features hypothesis or the surface account—has implications for clinical practice. For example, because the missing features perspective suggests a fundamental impairment in the underlying grammar of a child with SLI, it could be inferred that intervention should be oriented toward teaching compensatory strategies. However, if the problems of the child with SLI center on the processing of small, unstressed words and grammatical units, clinicians could address the problem by manipulating the input, by increasing the salience of the targeted grammatical form.

However, because available theories do not account for all patterns of strength and weakness, diverse and inclusive approaches to language intervention/clinical practice offer greater probability of success, particularly methods that incorporate general syntactic and semantic concerns. Four general suggestions for language facilitation practice and research are offered.

First, grammatical competencies are an important aspect of overall communicative competence, and as such, warrant a central place in intervention programming. In recent years, theoretic and practical emphasis in language intervention has shifted away from form toward use; with increasing focus on pragmatic aspects of the language system, such skills as initiating and responding in conversation have become intervention targets, at times, to the exclusion of grammatical emphases. Many positive changes in intervention and service delivery models have occurred because of this increased awareness of the central contribution of the social aspects of language, and without basic conversational abilities, grammatical competencies are not particularly powerful. However, it is limiting to overlook the integral relationship between the grammatical and social domains of linguistic competence.

The importance of making grammatical skills an intervention focus is supported by the fact that grammatical competencies prove to be a consistent and persistent problem for children with SLI. Current studies document that difficulties with particular aspects of the grammatical system can continue into adulthood (Records, Tomblin, & Freese, 1992; Tomblin, Freese, & Records, 1990). Furthermore, it is likely that grammatical skills serve both as the outgrowth of and agent for social interactive skills. Grammatical abilities are the medium through which social interactive aspects of language are accomplished. In turn, language interactions, and participation in them, informs the grammatical system (Fujiki & Brinton, chap. 8, this volume). Influence between domains is clearly bidirectional, and limitations in either dimension of language competence may impair development in the other. This perspective on the importance of the grammatical system is not incompatible with the current focus on facilitating linguistic skills in naturalistic environments via communicative interactions. Focus on language form, in conjunction with attention to aspects of language use, can occur within service delivery contexts and activities rooted in social interaction.

A second suggestion for language intervention is to center language input, models, and teaching strategies on the verb system. In facilitating grammar, results of the studies discussed here and elsewhere suggest that particular attention to the verb system is warranted (Rice, 1991). In brief, the notion is to use the verb as the centerpiece of grammatical intervention. By modeling main verb forms and building on children's use of verbs through recasts and expansion, not only is the verb form itself illustrated, but also the argument structures in which the verb participates, and the manner in which various grammatical inflections are associated with the form. Because many grammatical challenges seem to center on verbs and verb complements, approaching grammatical teaching from the perspective of highlighting the verb system should promote efficacy and efficiency in language facilitation. Thus, consideration should be given to enriching verb use in language input, as well as to illustrating the variety of inflections and argument structures allowable for a given verb form. For example, in a cooking activity, opportunity to emphasize the verb *stir* may occur. Highlighting the form within a range of syntactic frames and with several grammatical inflections (e.g., *She is stirring, She is stirring the dough, She stirs the dough, She stirs with a spoon, She is stirring quickly, She stirred the dough*) would seem to afford the greatest opportunity to enhance understanding and use of the verb and the associated inflections. It also seems likely that this type of verb-centered grammatical teaching will be most successfully built around activities in which the actual activities are occurring, with modeled language tied to real events and actions.

A third point for intervention is identifying emerging grammatical skills, and optimizing the timing of intervention emphases. As evidence builds for the genetic aspects of language impairments (Crago & Gopnik, chap. 3, this volume; Tomblin & Buckwalter, chap. 2, this volume), in conjunction with the finding that particular grammatical challenges can persist into adulthood, questions of when and how specific skills should be targeted take on particular significance. One key to advancing intervention science with respect to grammatical skills is to increase knowledge about the timing of intervention emphases, specifically, improving our ability to diagnose and recognize sensitive opportunities for grammatical facilitation. Identifying and targeting emerging grammatical skills (i.e., those with beginning patterns of mastery) should optimize intervention outcomes; however, our limited knowledge in recognizing emergent skills, particularly discerning when a skill requires intervention focus, and when it will develop independently, constrains our ability to optimize intervention timing. In addition, expanded knowledge of aspects of the grammatical system that seem to be particularly difficult to remediate, and those that seem more malleable, would be helpful.

The final suggestion for intervention involves the compelling need for clinicians and researchers to work toward perfecting treatment techniques. Additional study addressing the particulars of grammatically focused intervention is clearly warranted. It is appropriate for treatment research to move beyond the more basic questions of which intervention strategies can effect changes (because our available research literature suggests there are many; e.g., imitation, modeling, focused stimulation) toward more refined questions of which intervention strategies are particularly efficient and effective, yield maximal change over time and across settings, with particular linguistic competencies, and for which children.

In summary, grammatical problems are a key component of specific language impairment. Although a number of the grammatical features of the impairment have been identified, our understanding of how these features develop and change over time, why they are challenging, and how they relate to difficulties in other areas of the language system is less advanced. These challenges provide direction for our continued study, as motivated by both our drive to understand SLI and our need to provide appropriate intervention services to this population.

REFERENCES

Bolinger, D.L. (1971). *The phrasal verb in English*. Cambridge, MA: Harvard University Press.

Brown, R. (1973). *A first language*. Cambridge, MA: Harvard University Press.

Clahsen, H. (1989). The grammatical characterization of developmental dysphasia. *Linguistics, 27*, 987–920.

Clahsen, H. (1991). *Child language and developmental dysphasia*. Philadelphia: John Benjamins North America, Inc.

Clark, E.V., & Hecht, B.F. (1982). Learning to coin agent and instrument nouns. *Cognition, 12*, 1–24.

Dixon, R.M.W. (1982). The grammar of English phrasal verbs. *Australian Journal of Linguistics, 2*(1), 1–42.

Dunn, L.M., & Dunn, L.M. (1981). *Peabody Picture Vocabulary Test-Revised*. Circle Pines, MN: American Guidance Service.

Fletcher, P., & Peters, J. (1984). Characterizing language impairment in children: An exploratory study. *Language Testing, 1*, 33–49.

Fraser, B. (1976). *The verb particle combination in English*. New York: Academic Press.

Gleitman, L. (1989). The structural sources of verb meaning. *Papers and Reports on Child Language Development*. Stanford University Press, Stanford, CA.

Goodluck, H. (1986). Children's knowledge of prepositional phrase structure: An experimental test. *Journal of Psycholinguistic Research, 15*, 177–188.

Gopnik, M., & Crago, M. (1991). Familial aggregation of a developmental language disorder. *Cognition, 39*, 1–50.

Johnston, J.R., & Schery, T. (1976). The use of grammatical morphemes by children with communication disorders. In D. Morehead & A. Morehead (Eds.), *Normal and deficient child language* (pp. 239–258). Baltimore, MD: University Park Press.

Khan, L., & James, S. (1983). Grammatical morpheme development in three language disordered children. *Journal of Childhood Communication Disorders, 6*, 85–100.

Lahey, M., Liebergott, J., Chesnick, M., Menyuk, P., & Adams, J. (1992). Variability in the use of grammatical morphemes: Implications for understanding language impairment. *Applied Psycholinguistics, 13*, 373–398.

Leonard, L.B. (1988). Lexical development and processing in specific language impairment. In R.L. Schiefelbusch & L.L. Lloyd (Eds.), *Language perspectives: Acquisition, retardation, and intervention* (2nd ed., pp. 69–87). Austin, TX: PRO-ED.

Leonard, L.B. (1989). Language learnability and specific language impairment in children. *Applied Psycholinguistics, 10*, 179–202.

Leonard, L.B., Bortolini, U., Caselli, M.C., McGregor, K.K., & Sabbadini, L. (1992). Two accounts of morphological deficits in children with specific language impairment. *Language Acquisition, 2*, 151–179.

Pinker, S. (1984). *Language learnability and language acquisition*. Cambridge, MA: Harvard University Press.

Pinker, S. (1989). *Learnability and cognition: The acquisition of argument structure*. Cambridge, MA: Harvard University Press.

Quirk, R., Greenbaum, S., Leech, G., & Svartvik, J. (1985). *A comprehensive grammar of the English language*. London: Longman Publishing Group.

Records, N.L., Tomblin, J.B., & Freese, P.R. (1992). The quality of life of young adults with histories of specific language impairment. *American Journal of Speech-Language Pathology, 1*, 44–53.

Rice, M.L. (1991). Children with specific language impairment: Toward a model of teachability. In N. Krasnegor, D.M. Rumbaugh, R.L. Schiefelbusch, & M. Studdert-Kennedy (Eds.), *Biological and behavioral determinants of language development* (pp. 447–480). Hillsdale, NJ: Lawrence Erlbaum Associates.

Rice, M.L., & Bode, J.V. (1993). GAPS in the verb lexicons of children with specific language impairment. *First Language, 13*, 113–131.

Rice, M.L., Buhr, J.C., & Nemeth, M.J. (1990). Fast mapping word learning abilities of language delayed preschoolers. *Journal of Speech and Hearing Disorders, 55*, 33–42.

Rice, M.L., & Oetting, J.B. (1991, October). *Morphological deficits of SLI children: Evaluation of number marking and agreement*. Paper presented at the Boston University Conference on Language Development, Boston.

Steckol, K., & Leonard, L.B. (1979). The use of grammatical morphemes by normal and language-impaired children. *Journal of Communication Disorders, 12,* 291–301.

Tomblin, J.B., Freese, P.R., & Records, N.L. (1990, June). *Language, cognitive, and social characteristics of young adults with histories of developmental language disorder.* Paper presented at the Symposium on Research in Child Language Disorders, Madison, WI.

Watkins, R.V., Buhr, J.C., & Davis, C. (submitted). *Acquisition of one derivational morpheme by children with specific language impairment.*

Watkins, R.V., & Rice, M.L. (1991). Verb particle and preposition acquisition in language-impaired preschoolers. *Journal of Speech and Hearing Research, 34,* 1130–1141.

Watkins, R.V., Rice, M.L., & Moltz, C.C. (1993). Verb use by language-impaired and normally developing children. *First Language, 13,* 133–143.

5

Grammatical Categories of Children with Specific Language Impairments

Mabel L. Rice

THE CONDITION OF INTEREST IN this chapter, as elsewhere in this volume, is that of specific language impairment (SLI). This condition is defined operationally as evident in individuals who demonstrate all the prerequisites for language acquisition, such as adequate intellectual ability, intact auditory acuity, neuromotor mechanisms free from defect, and socioemotional competency, but who, nevertheless, demonstrate difficulties with language acquisition. Advances in what we know about this condition have led to a reformulation of how we think about the grammatical limitations of individuals who demonstrate SLI (for reviews of the literature, see Bishop, 1992; Johnston, 1988; Leonard, 1989; Rice, 1991). Many scholars now view SLI as a possible long-term impairment, one that persists into adulthood. It seems to be a longstanding condition, rather than a temporary delay in the onset of language milestones, although the surface symptoms change over time. It is important to note that this is viewed as a likely language impairment in adulthood, not merely a language-turned-reading-impairment, as school-age learning disabilities can be regarded. Another major change in our understanding of this disorder is the recognition that individuals affected with SLI tend to cluster within families (cf. Tomblin & Buckwalter, chap. 2, and Crago & Gopnik, chap. 3, this volume). This finding leads to a reconsideration of possible etiological factors in a way that includes a plausible role for genetic mechanisms of transmission. Finally, another and very significant rethinking is that

I would like to acknowledge the contributions of Ken Wexler. Collaborative work with Ken has shaped much of my understanding of the linguistic frameworks herein. His encouragement of my efforts and his assistance in working out the formulations of the Spec, head, and Optional Infinitive accounts of SLI are greatly appreciated. Whatever inaccuracies and errors of interpretation evident in this paper are my own. I also wish to recognize the assistance of my students, Janna Oetting, Soyeong Pae, and Pat Cleave, as well as Mary Howe, Research Associate, with data analyses and interpretation.

with regard to the nature of the language deficit. At issue is where to place the locus of the problem. One dominant view has been a language delay account, in which SLI is viewed as difficulty with some general learning mechanism that initiates the process of language acquisition. Alternative views have focused on processing limitations, in which SLI is thought to be a particular problem with processing the input stream of spoken language. More recently, limited linguistic mechanisms have been proposed, in which selective deficits in the underlying mental representations of linguistic structures are postulated.

This chapter addresses the issue of how to characterize the nature of the language deficit exhibited by children with SLI. The topics are presented in the following order. First is a synopsis of three interpretations of the morphological deficits of children with SLI, highlighting the significance of two English morphemes—regular plurals and verb agreement. Following that is a more detailed discussion of what is involved in the use of these morphemes. Next is a description of recent findings obtained in our laboratory of how children with SLI perform on these morphemes. After identifying some interesting details of the acquisition patterns, a functional categories account of morphosyntax is introduced. This perspective is then applied to the data available from children with SLI, with the identification of two new linguistic accounts of morphological deficits. After that, the competing models are re-evaluated, followed by a discussion of future research directions and clinical implications.

I argue that there is much to be gained by close scrutiny of grammatical particulars and associated theoretical models. At the same time, I also recognize, and have argued elsewhere, that the surface manifestations of difficulties with language acquisition can and do cut across other language dimensions. Word acquisition is often vulnerable (cf. Rice, Buhr, & Nemeth, 1990; Rice, Buhr, & Oetting, 1992; Rice, Cleave, Oetting, & Pae, 1993; Rice, Oetting, Marquis, Bode, & Pae, in press), including limited verb lexicons (cf. Rice & Bode, 1993). Phonological deficits are often concomitant symptoms. Furthermore, the relation between language impairment and social competence is intricate and clinically very significant (cf. Gertner, Hadley, & Rice, 1993; Hadley & Rice, 1991; Rice, 1993 a, b; Rice, Hadley, & Alexander, in press; Rice, Sell, & Hadley, 1991).

Full understanding of SLI will require, ultimately, a model that can reasonably integrate these dimensions. That goal rather surpasses the robustness of current models, however. Until such time as comprehensive models are viable, then, work must proceed on multiple, but somewhat separate, fronts if we are to arrive at a full characterization of specific language impairment. It may be that more than one "problem" is evident, with more than one "cause," or, alternatively, that some surface problems derive from other underlying problems, or, possibly, the various surface manifestations are all part of the same underlying faulty mechanisms or acquisition processes.

At the same time, morphology is a well-documented locus of difficulty for individuals with SLI, and any successful account of this condition must be able to predict the specific problems in this area. Thus, detailed descriptions of morphological competencies are essential for characterizing the nature of the deficits. There are also some clearly articulated and competing hypotheses about the source of morphological difficulties. Thus, this is an area of work where it is possible to bring a theoretical perspective to empirical evidence, and, conversely, to bring evidence to theoretical claims.

THREE INTERPRETATIONS OF MORPHOLOGICAL DEFICITS

Three current interpretations of the morphological deficits of children with SLI are of interest here. The models differ in the status of the language mechanisms attributed to the child, the locus of the problem, and predicted patterns of morphological deficit. These models, and related predictions, are summarized in Table 1.

Delayed Language

Advocates of this account (cf. Curtiss, Katz, & Tallal, 1992; Lahey, Liebergott, Chesnick, Menyuk, & Adams, 1992) conclude that children with SLI do not show unusual grammars or specific difficulties with particular morphemes. Instead, their language is simply slower in development. This Delayed Language model has been evident in the literature since the earliest studies. Adherents to this position argue that there is no difference between the grammar of children with SLI and that of younger, linguistically matched, typically developing children. Thus, the language mechanisms of SLI are regarded as similar to those of typically developing children, but, for unspecified reasons, they are late in activating and/or they require a longer period of time for completion. The distinction between onset and rate of acquisition mechanisms versus underlying linguistic representations is a useful one, in that it is plausible that acquisition mechanisms could be implicated at the same time that underlying structures could be sound. Another valuable contribution of this model is the designation of a language-equivalent normative comparison group as the relevant reference group. This comparison has come to constitute the null hypothesis for studies of the grammar of children with SLI. The prediction of the Delayed Language model for morphology is that children with SLI should not differ from a comparison group of younger language-matched children. However, demonstration of group differences offers strong evidence of focal areas of linguistic deficiencies. Thus, the prediction for the two English morphemes of interest here, regular plurals and verb agreement, is that the mean accuracy levels for the children in the SLI group should not differ from those of the normal comparison group.

Table 1. Models of morphological deficits

Model	Status of linguistic mechanism	Locus of the problem	Relevant comparisons	Predicted outcomes (English morphology)
Language Delay	Intact	Delayed onset; faulty rate of acquisition mechanisms	SLI = Language equivalent (LE) SLI < Chronological age (CA)	General delay; morphological profile corresponds to normal acquisition. For plurals and agreement, SLI = LE
Surface Account	Intact learning mechanisms but incomplete representations	Morphophonological; unstressed bound and closed class morphemes are systematically filtered from the input	SLI < LE SLE < CA	Omissions of certain unstressed morphemes For regular plurals and subject/verb agreement marking, bare stems
Limited Linguistic Mechanisms/Structures	Selective deficits	Morphosyntactic; morphology as manifestation of syntactic relations and principles	SLI < LE SLI < CA	Difficulties with clusters of syntactically related morphemes 1) Missing Agreement: for plurals, SLI = LE; for agreement, SLI < LE 2) Missing Feature: for plurals and agreement, SLI < LE 3) Spec, head:[a] Plurals: SLI = LE for Det + noun; SLI < LE for quantifier + noun Agreement: SLI < LE 4) Optional infinitive:[a] for plurals, no prediction; for agreement, SLI < LE

[a]Introduced in this chapter.

Surface Account

One way in which the mechanisms of language acquisition could be impaired is an inability to process the incoming stream of speech. Several versions of this possibility have been proposed, with some models operative at basic levels of perception (e.g., Tallal & Piercy, 1973) and others more concerned with the grammatical level of interpretation. The one of interest here, because it is the most explicitly developed and relevant to the evidence, is the Surface Account, put forth by Leonard (1989; Leonard, chap. 6 this volume; Leonard, Bortolini, Caselli, McGregor, & Sabbadini, 1992). This account is motivated by the conclusion that children with SLI, relative to their language-matched peers, have problems with a subset of morphemes, the unstressed bound and closed class morphemes. This difficulty is attributed to a systematic distortion of the input, so that the ability to form grammatical paradigms is hampered by a limited access to the morphological information in the input. The problem is regarded as morphophonemic in nature (i.e., a problem in processing the surface [phonetic] realization of morphological units). The underlying linguistic acquisition mechanisms are thought to be intact, but the formation of linguistic representations (grammatical paradigms) are incomplete; children with SLI can be regarded as normal language learners who must compensate for input that is distorted in certain ways. For the two morphemes discussed here, the prediction put forth by Leonard et al. is that the -*s* affix, as a nonstressed, unsalient morpheme, will be more difficult for English-speaking children with SLI than for their language-matched peers. This prediction holds for plurals and verb agreement marking. An additional prediction is that the form of morphological deficit is that of zero markings (i.e., omission of targeted forms). These predictions correspond to the conventional clinical impressions of children with SLI, as children who are likely to have problems with the production of grammatical morphemes, and who tend to omit the little, unstressed, functional grammatical markers.

Limited Linguistic Mechanisms

Another interpretation focuses on the underlying linguistic structures, and postulates that the source of disruption is to be found in the linguistic mechanisms available to the children. These children, then, face the language acquisition process with selective deficits in the linguistic framework that supports normal acquisition. This model has been advocated by Clahsen (1989, 1992), who concluded that German-speaking children with SLI have particular difficulty establishing agreement relations, presumably because they lack or do not fully utilize a Control Agreement Principle (Clahsen, 1992, henceforth referred to as Missing Agreement Control). Another version of a limited linguistic mechanisms account has been put forth by Gopnik (1990) and Gopnik and Crago (1991). In these accounts, individuals with SLI are said to be missing abstract syntactic–semantic features (henceforth the Missing Features Model). These features were thought to be marked on each lexical item, and to trigger related morphological rules. The claim was that the affected individuals were missing feature-marking for the features of number, gender, animacy, mass/count, proper names, tense, and aspect. For example, number marking on the noun would be needed for plural marking. The concept of plurality could be available as a semantic notion, but would not be marked for morphological expression. The relevant prediction, then, is that neither plurals nor agreement would be marked correctly, because of the missing feature of number, which is essential for both.

It is important to note the contrast between the limited linguistic mechanisms perspective and the previous accounts. The level of analysis shifts significantly from the surface properties of morphemes to underlying linguistic representations or mechanisms. In turn, following the tenets of contemporary linguistic theory, the linguistic mechanisms are thought to be part of a universal grammar that is under the direct control of genetic mechanisms. Thus, it is plausible to predict a pattern of familial involvement that is consistent with known mechanisms of genetic transmission. Therefore, this model puts the problem squarely in language-specific deficits that are likely to be inherited.

I argue that this model warrants full consideration. The predictions of the two accounts reviewed so far, those of Missing Agreement Control and Missing Feature, differ somewhat in that the former predicts selective impairment of agreement marking but not plurals, whereas the latter predicts difficulties with both.

ENGLISH REGULAR PLURALS AND VERB AGREEMENT

Consider what is involved in the use of English regular plurals and verb agreement marking. The two morphemes share the same surface form (if we ignore some allomorphic variations), a form that is unstressed and of low phonetic salience. So both are vulnerable for input processing (cf. Leonard et al., 1992). But the linguistic functions of the two morphemes differ.

For the plurals, we restrict our analysis to count nouns, the names of things such as *dog* and *cat,* and the regular plural marking, the *-s* affix. The plural carries a referential assignment, that of referring to numerosity. *Dog* means a single dog; *dogs* refers to more than one dog. There is reason to believe that even young children with SLI do not have trouble with the semantics of plurals (i.e., they seem to know the difference between one and more than one thing, and use terms such as *lots of* to indicate plurality). The question is whether they can convert that knowledge into linguistic form, to mark plurality on the noun. Henceforth, number marking is referred to as NUM; + NUM indicates plural contexts; and − NUM singular. Note that full control of NUM marking requires *selectivity* of application; that is, selecting the appropriate form class, marking NUM on nouns only. It also requires *contrastivity;* that is, marking NUM as + only in cases of plurality and not in cases of singularity. Finally, as children learn the rules for NUM marking, they may *overgeneralize* this rule to exceptional cases, such as *mans* and *fishes*. Thus, *selectivity, contrastivity,* and *overgeneralization* can serve as linguistic criteria for mastery of NUM. Much of the current literature about plural acquisition, and the competencies of children with SLI, have focused on these levels of NUM marking.

Another kind of marking is relevant at linguistic levels beyond the noun, and is relevant for understanding the nature of the grammatical representations of children with SLI. NUM marking must *agree* with other information in the noun phrase and the verb phrase. Articles are marked for NUM and this marking must agree with the noun NUM. Thus, *a dog* or *this dog* shows agreement, as does *these dogs,* but **these dog* or **a dogs* does not. Also, in English, numerical quantifiers are marked for NUM and must agree with the noun NUM marking. Thus, *one dog* or *two dogs* shows agreement, but not **one dogs* or **two dog.*

Verbs can be marked for tense (unlike nouns), person (a nonreferential linguistic marking), and NUM. The class of verbs of interest here are the matrix, or lexicalized, verbs that can serve as main verbs in a sentence (e.g., *walk*). So, in English, the final *-s* morpheme (e.g., *he walks*), marks present tense, third person, and singular. The final *-s* is also thought to be marked for agreement, in that the person and NUM markings must agree with the person and NUM markings on the subject. Thus, *he goes* is acceptable, but **he go* or **they goes* is not, nor is **I goes* allowed.

EVIDENCE FROM ENGLISH-SPEAKING CHILDREN WITH SLI

The evidence reported here is drawn from a study of 50 English-speaking 5-year-old children with SLI. These children's spontaneous language productions were compared to those of a comparison group of 58 younger, typically developing children of equivalent mean length of utterance, whose mean age was 38 months. Because the study is reported in considerable detail elsewhere (Rice & Oetting, 1993), the description here highlights the key findings relevant to the subsequent discussion.

The procedures consisted of computer-assisted transcript analyses, which proceeded in phases. First, a summary measure of the mean percent correct in obligatory contexts was calculated for each group, and the group performance levels were compared. For plurals, the means for the two groups were: SLI, 83%; language-matched comparison, 93%. This difference is statistically significant, $p < .01$. For third person singular marking on the verb, the means were: SLI, 36%; language-matched group, 54%, also statistically significant, $p < .01$.

At first glance, then, the findings do not support the Delayed Language account (because of the better performance of the control group for both morphemes, a finding not predicted by this model). However, the group means are consistent with the predictions of the Surface Account. Relative to their language-equivalent peers, the SLI group had lower overall performance on the two unstressed morphemes. Yet the mean performance levels for the plurals are quite high for the SLI group, at or near conventional levels of mastery, suggesting that plural acquisition may be more robust than indicated by a simple group comparison.

In order to evaluate the children's plural acquisition further, the transcripts were examined for evidence of *selectivity, contrastivity,* and *overgeneralizations.* A further criteria, that of *productivity,* was measured by tallying the number of different nouns marked for NUM. The findings are as follows.

Both groups marked NUM on multiple noun stems, and neither group had problems with selectivity (NUM marking appeared on nouns and not other form classes). Children in the SLI group, as well as children in the control group, made creative errors of overregularization, such as *mans* and *herselves.* The contrastivity analyses also revealed similarities between the groups. The transcripts were searched for instances of misapplications of plurals to singular nouns (i.e., *toys* when the referent was one toy). There were such errors in both groups, although the overall rates were low (2.6% for SLI, 3.2% for MLU matches). However, the groups did differ in the other form of contrastivity error, that of zero marking for plurals (i.e., *toy* for *toys*). For the SLI group, the average percent of zero marking per child was 16% (53/404); for the MLU matches, these errors were evident in 7% of the nouns (38/473), a statistically significant difference ($p < .01$).

What are we to make of these findings? On some indices, the SLI group seems to have control of NUM markings on nouns. The overregularizations are presumptive evidence of rule acquisition; + NUM affixes are restricted to nouns, and appear on multiple nouns; and + NUM markings are seldom misapplied to − NUM nouns. (In a subsequent study by Oetting & Rice [1993], with independent samples of 5-year-old children with SLI and control groups of typically developing children, the finding of robust use of plurals by affected children is replicated for plural affixation and observed further in noun compounding tasks.) The problem seems to be with the − NUM markings on the nouns, the bare stems with omitted affixes. What is happening here?

The answer to that question requires consideration of agreement marking on the noun. Inspection of the transcripts revealed that the − NUM occurrences depended upon the configuration of the components within the noun phrase. Concordance listings were generated of all instances of plural marking and coded plural errors (including bare stems), and coded errors with articles. Almost all the instances of − NUM could be classified into one of two categories. One was that of determiner/noun, as in *those bottle. The other was that of numerical quantifier, as in *two bottle. Errors appeared in the transcripts of both groups of children. An overall error rate was calculated by searching for the following determiners, *a, an, this, that, these, those, every,* and *some* and the following numerical quantifiers, *one, two, three, four, five,* and *nine,* and determining a mean percent correct use in obligatory contexts. The determiner contexts did not differentiate the two groups. SLI and language equivalent children were both very accurate in this context, with 96% correct for children with SLI and 97% for MLU-matched children. However, the groups did differ in the quantifier contexts. The mean for the SLI group was 71%, whereas the language control children were 90% accurate.

Is it the case that the differences in the quantifier contexts account for the group differences in the overall summary of percent correct of plurals? To evaluate this possibility, the summary means were recalculated, without the quantifier contexts. For the SLI group, the mean percentage correct raised to 86%, and the MLU group raised to 94%. The difference between the groups dropped out of the conventional p levels for reliability, with a p value of .09.

What can we make of this? NUM marking seems to be vulnerable in ways not predicted by either the phonetic salience of the surface realization of the morpheme, or of the NUM marking itself. Obviously, if children with SLI can mark NUM accurately by affixing the -*s* to nouns in the 634 out of 660 times when it is preceded by a determiner, they do not seem to be having significant problems with either the affix or the notion of NUM. So what is the locus of the difficulty? The problems with verb agreement suggest that agreement marking may be implicated. Is there reason to believe that there are underlying linguistic similarities between English verb agreement and quantifier + noun agreement that would introduce complexities for children with SLI in a way that is different from that of determiner/noun agreement? Current models of morphosyntax suggest that could be the case.

FUNCTIONAL CATEGORIES

Functional categories are elaborations of X-bar syntactic theory (cf. Haegemann, 1991; Radford, 1990). Within this view of syntax, phrase structures are thought to be headed by the lexical categories of nouns, verbs, adjectives, or prepositions. To use the noun phrase (NP) as an example, nouns are heads, which can then be expanded (projected) to a higher level of phrase structure.

For example, the noun phrase "that peanut in the cup" can be represented in the following way:

NP
det   N'
              |
              N

that   peanut in the cup

In this case, "peanut" is the head for the NP, and "in the cup" is a complement that expands it to a next higher level, that of N'. The determiner in this representation adjoins to the N'. The NP is regarded as the maximal projection for the N. Recently, it has been proposed that the determiner is also a head, of what is called a "functional" (i.e., nonlexical) category, which can also project to a higher, maximal level. (The determiner category consists of *a/the/this/that/some/any/no/much,* cf. Radford, 1990.) This can be represented as follows:

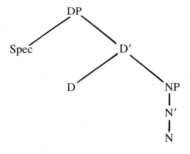

just   that   peanut in the cup

In this example, there is an additional position for the Specifier, which adjoins to the D' level. (Specifiers are defined in this relational way [i.e., as sisters to an X', where X can stand for any head].) Notice that the determiner (that) is in a head position (D) and so is the noun (peanut; N).

It is thought that this general schema applies to all four kinds of lexical heads, to generate NPs, verb phrases (VPs), adjective phrases (APs), and prepositional phrases (PPs). Similarly, the notion of functional categories has been extended to other parts of the grammar. These functional categories share several characteristics. They constitute closed classes, they are generally phonologically and morphologically dependent, and unstressed; they mark grammatical or relational features, rather than picking out a class of objects (Radford, 1990, p. 53). In the VP, separate nodes are now identified for *complementizers* (words that introduce complement clauses, such as *that/for/whether/if*), *agreement,* and *tense.*

Contemporary linguistic theory is concerned with how to configure the functional categories and with the underlying mechanisms and principles. Within these models, inflections are treated as interacting with deeply syntactic processes. The claim is that processes of head movement (where verbs are considered to be heads) are deeply interwoven with inflection. According to Wexler (1992, p. 6) "Thus to ask whether a child knows the processes governing inflection is, in part, to ask whether a child knows head movement, . . . and processes controlling head movement."

Consider a current model of agreement (cf. Chomsky, 1992). The configuration is as follows:

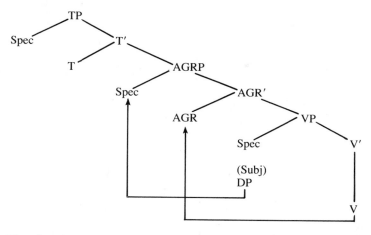

The gist of the interpretation is that the subject is generated in the Spec of the V', and must move to Spec, AGR, so it can be checked for agreement. The verb moves to AGR to be checked for agreement. The checking is carried out at the level of number and person features marked on the verb and the noun, and must conform to certain principles of the grammar.

FUNCTIONAL CATEGORIES
PERSPECTIVES ON THE MORPHOLOGY OF SLI

An elaborated X-bar schema allows for several important generalizations to be made about the grammar of children with SLI. In our samples from English-speaking children with SLI, lexical heads do not seem to be problematic for children with SLI, nor are the fundamental configurational relations (i.e., word order within constituents generally is not disturbed [although there may be vulnerability in certain contexts requiring verb movement]; also reported by Clahsen, 1992, to be true for German-speaking children with SLI).

In some broadly defined ways, then, the grammar of individuals with SLI can be thought to follow the configurational constraints evident in universal grammar.

At a more detailed linguistic level, though, the grammar does not seem to be so robust. Consider, now, the details that were reported earlier about plural and agreement marking of the affected children. Recall that they seem to have + NUM marking worked out for nouns in the *determiner + noun* context, but not completely so for the *quantifier + noun,* and they have considerable difficulty with agreement marking on the verb.

Spec, Head Agreement

On the model of functional categories sketched out above, we can see that the derivation of correct subject–verb agreement involves a process of Spec, head agreement. Another observation can also be drawn, that the Determiner, noun agreement occurs at the level of Head, head relation, although the details of how the agreement checking would work are not, as far as I know, worked out well for English NPs. These observations accord well with the evidence that -*s* agreement at the clause level is less consistently marked by children with SLI than for the control group, whereas plural markings (especially the *Det + noun* context) are at or near mastery for both groups. Thus, configurational differences within the functional categories accord with observed differences across morphemes with the same surface forms, so that Spec, head agreement marking is affected but Head, head plural marking is not.

If these configurational relations are significant factors in the vulnerabilities in the grammar of children with SLI, it suggests that one characteristic of SLI grammar may be that of particular problems with agreement relations at the level of Spec, head. If so, the observed deficit in performance within the NP, in the *quantifier + noun* context (assuming that these differences are reliable and hold up empirically, which certainly needs to be established) implicates a specifier position for the quantifier within the NP. Such details are not yet available for the agreement relations with the NP, and it remains to be seen if this possibility can be established.

A prediction that follows from the Spec, head interpretation is that other Spec, head relations should also be vulnerable. There is evidence available in support of this prediction. Within the model advanced by Chomsky (1992), case assignment on the noun is checked in the Spec position in the NP. Thus, if Spec, head relations are problematic for children with SLI, then case should also be affected. That prediction is borne out by evidence reported by Loeb and Leonard (1991), who found that English-speaking children with SLI showed difficulty with case marking on pronouns, relative to a language-equivalent control group. Similarly, Clahsen (1992) reports problems with case-marking for German-speaking children with SLI.

It must be noted that this account of agreement-marking limitations differs in some important ways from Clahsen's model of a deficit Control Agreement Principle (cf. Clahsen, 1992), in that his model predicts difficulty with determiners and adjectives, a prediction which, according to his report, holds for German-speaking children with SLI. On the Spec, head interpretation as sketched above, determiners are thought to be a Head, head relation. In the evidence presented here for English-speaking children with SLI, the agreement checking between determiners and plurals is not problematic (although there is evidence that determiners may be more likely to be omitted by these children, but this may be for reasons other than agreement). Under the Spec, head account, these differences could be resolved if it proves to be the case that the determiners for which agreement marking is difficult for German-speaking children with SLI are located in Spec rather than in the head of DP. That possibility remains to be seen.

All things considered, the Spec, head account offers a reasonably plausible way to capture the empirical evidence from English-speaking children with SLI (i.e., that the same surface form [-s], carries agreement, but this agreement marking plays out differently within the NP and the VP, so that the condition of SLI involves selective deficits with the latter but not the former). There are, however, other possible perspectives with regard to -s agreement marking that also have high potential value for interpretation of SLI.

Optional Infinitives

Working within the linguistic framework laid out above, Wexler (1992) has proposed that omitted -s for third person contexts, which young, typically developing English-speaking children tend to do, can be regarded as an optional use of the infinitival form. Because in English the infinitival form of the verb is the bare stem also used in simple present tense for all but third person, infinitival forms are not clearly distinguishable from finite (i.e., tense-marked) verb forms. Given the sparse surface morphology of English, much of the evidence in support of this hypothesis comes from other languages in which infinitival forms are more evident, such as French and German. What is relevant here is that the hypothesis claims that there is an initial period in which typically developing children optionally add -s to mark agreement, and that this period is resolved when children master tense marking. When youngsters say, *he go, it is interpreted as a selection of the default form of the verb, the infinitival form. The choice of the infinitive is considered optional, on this view, because the children do not understand tense, which in English would be evident by incomplete or inaccurate marking of past tense in utterances such as he walked, which are likely to appear as *he walk.

On this view, then, several new directions emerge for accounts of SLI (see Rice & Wexler, 1993, for an elaborated discussion of this model). One consequence is that the notion of "delayed language" takes on a more specific interpretation. Within an Optional Infinitive model, the finding that children with SLI have selective difficulty with -s agreement could be because they remain longer in a period in which the bare stems (i.e., infinitival forms) are regarded as optional, a period that other children pass through at an earlier MLU level. The findings reported above for the SLI group, then, could be viewed as a simple delay in the acquisition of plurals, at least within the determiner + plural context (i.e., with underlying representations similar to that of children at equivalent MLU levels). However, the acquisition of agreement demonstrates a not-so-simple delay, in which the expected period of optionality extends far beyond that demonstrated by unaffected individuals.

Two other important predictions for the grammar of children with SLI follow from the Optional Infinitive account. One is that the period of optional agreement marking for the children with SLI will be contemporaneous with problems with tense marking (a prediction borne out for children with SLI, cf. Leonard et al., 1992). A second prediction is that the onset of agreement mastery will be preceded by the acquisition of tense marking. This is a rather strong prediction, in that it posits a direct relation between two morphemes that have different surface forms and mark different grammatical functions that are nevertheless linked in the grammatical system. Furthermore, the correct way to test the prediction is to evaluate the relative levels of acquisition of the morphemes for individual children. The relevant evidence, then, is to be drawn from observations of individuals, where considerable variability is known to occur (cf. Lahey et al., 1992).

In evidence collected in our laboratory, we find support for this prediction. In an elicitation task, children produced regular past tense (e.g., *walked*), and third person singular agreement (e.g., *walks*). There were 20 children in each of three groups: SLI, language-equivalent (MLU), and age-equivalent (CA). The analysis included children who demonstrated at least five obligatory contexts for both grammatical forms. After application of this criterion, 19 children in the SLI group remained, 12 in the MLU group, and 22 in the CA group. Of the SLI group, 11 children showed floor level performance on both morphemes, 2 showed equivalent performances on both, 5 demonstrated the predicted better performance on tense marking, whereas 1 demonstrated better performance on agreement marking. For the MLU group, the number of children in parallel categories was as follows: four for mastery on both, two for floor level on both, four children demonstrated the predicted difference, and two demonstrated the nonpredicted difference. For the CA group, 18 children were at mastery level for both, 1 child was at equivalent but not mastery for both morphemes, 1 demonstrated the predicted difference, and 2 the nonpredicted difference. Assuming that joint mastery, joint floor effects, and equivalent performance are consistent with the predicted pattern, as well as cases where both morphemes are at intermediate levels and tense is more accurately marked (by more than 10 percentage points) than agreement, 18 of the SLI children conformed to the pattern, as did 10 of the MLU group and 20 of the CA group. What this suggests is that at least this aspect of the grammatical system of children with SLI (i.e., the interrelation of tense and agreement) follows the same general principles that characterize the language acquisition of children without SLI, but the particular mechanisms that activate tense marking may be more vulnerable for the affected children.

Re-evaluation of the Competing Models of Morphological Deficits

How well do the models outlined in Table 1 account for the evidence presented above, for the plural and agreement morphemes of English-speaking children with SLI? The key empirical predictions target the comparison between children with SLI and their language-equivalent peers, where a lower performance on the part of the children with SLI can be viewed as a difficulty not fully accounted for by a delayed acquisition onset and, therefore, as presumptive evidence of potential deficits in an underlying linguistic acquisition mechanism. The predicted outcomes posited by the models are only partially met. For the Language Delay model, the predicted competence with plurals is observed (although the observed difference in plural contexts is not accounted for), but this account does not hold for agreement. For the Surface Account, the picture is reversed: the predicted problems with plurals are not evident, although the predicted agreement problem is confirmed. For the Missing Agreement account, the difficulty with verbal agreement is as predicted, but the apparent difference in plural marking within the NP (between determiner + noun contexts and quantifier + nouns) is unforeseen. The Missing Feature account's postulation of missing number marking, which in turn is responsible for missing agreement marking, is jeopardized by evidence that the children with SLI control number marking.

In order to illuminate more of the underlying grammar of children with SLI, a model was described in which morphemes are viewed as maximal projections of phrase structures, as functional (i.e., nonlexical) categories. In this model, ways in which plurals share properties with -s agreement are apparent, as well as ways in which the configurational properties differ. This led to the formulation of a Spec, head account, which also—and accurately—predicts problems with case marking for children with SLI.

A second model within a functional categories perspective was introduced, that of Optional Infinitives. This model provides an elaborated account of the observed missing agreement marking that brings the added advantages of accurately predicting problems with tense marking, and in specifying a crucial antecedent condition for mastery of agreement (i.e., mastery of tense).

It is much too early to predict the final fate of these new models of the grammatical limitations of individuals affected with SLI. The linguistic formulations are new, many of the particulars remain to be worked out, and the specific details are complex. What is clear, however, even at these early stages of inquiry, is the need to refine further the rather broadly drawn explanations of SLI, such as those embodied by a "delayed" versus "deficit" dichotomy. What is of primary interest is how to characterize the underlying language acquisition mechanisms and the representations of the grammar of SLI. Emerging evidence from detailed linguistic observations suggests that the story is likely to be rather more complicated, and more interesting, than a simple either/or choice would allow.

FUTURE RESEARCH GUIDELINES

If we are to come to understand the nature of language impairment, we can conclude from the previous discussion that we must arrive at a judicious mix of careful empirical documentation of the relevant phenomena, in particular, the ways in which the linguistic forms and structures of individuals with SLI differ from the expected ones, and devise theoretically motivated tests of predicted outcomes. In particular, it is essential that a well-grounded model of language serve as a guide to the formulation of testable hypotheses.

If there is to be continued momentum in our understanding of the morphological deficits of SLI, we must find ways to maintain high empirical standards, at the same time that we move toward more refined theoretical models. In the interest of formulating sound research guidelines, the following suggestions are offered:

1. The linguistic competencies of individuals with SLI must be documented in careful empirical detail. Although such details are accumulating in the literature, many, many more remain to be identified and documented. Our research efforts are doomed to failure if we overlook crucial distinctions.

2. We can benefit from continued use of the comparative group design, in which a language-equivalent group serves as a normative control. This is because this design generates valuable indices of central tendencies and individual variability, which are absolutely essential for the formulation of empirically sound generalizations that are likely to be reliable.

3. At the same time, group analyses alone are not sufficient. Detailed linguistic analyses must be carried out at the level of individual grammars, and predicted outcomes must be verifiable in individual linguistic profiles. In this age of morpheme-by-morpheme computer-generated calculations of mean percent correct in obligatory contexts, it must be pointed out that such summary figures can be misleading. The example here is that plural marking is more complex than just NUM marking. The vulnerable aspects of plural marking, if they exist for SLI grammars, may be at the level of agreement relations, which are thought to be located in the morphosyntax, not at the level of feature-marking on individual words. In a similar manner, counts of correct occurrences of the use of auxiliary BE forms summed across all

contexts can obscure very important differences in how they are used by children with SLI (cf. Hadley, 1993).

4.   Linguistic models that predict relations among morphemes and syntax have the potential for revealing what is spared and what is affected in the grammar of people with SLI. A primary advantage of such models, as demonstrated here, is the ability to generate specific questions that align with the symptomatology of SLI, questions that are testable and can, thereby, contribute to the evaluation of competing explanations.

5.   It is important to continue to explore the differentiation between processing mechanisms (cf. Johnston, chap. 7, this volume; Leonard, chap. 6, this volume) and underlying mental representations of grammar, insofar as these are conceptually distinct sources of potential dysfunction.

6.   In modern inquiry it is essential to consider language-specific aspects of SLI, or, conversely, the linguistic universals manifest or missing in SLI (cf. Clahsen, 1992; Leonard, chap. 6, this volume).

7.   Finally, there must be a way to connect the observed areas of linguistic difficulty with the emerging reports of familial aggregation of affected individuals. An obvious advantage of the functional categories account outlined here is that, for independent reasons, adherents of this view argue that there are universal configurations of morphosyntax, which are part of the innate endowment of the human language capacity. If there is, in fact, an inherited language capacity, it is plausible that certain mechanisms or structures could be vulnerable for individuals with SLI. Such a claim has the admirable virtue of linking the surface symptomology of SLI with the underlying etiology. The significance of this claim calls for full evaluation.

CLINICAL IMPLICATIONS

By now, some readers might be wondering if the usefulness of these analyses and observations is limited to the conclusion that scientists spend too much time poring over transcripts. Much of this inquiry, however, is motivated by the conviction that the research efforts will culminate in clinically significant outcomes. These are apparent when we consider the following three areas of clinical endeavor. ⸱

Identification

The identification of individuals with SLI remains a vexing clinical issue. The standard assessment batteries are not particularly sensitive to targeted areas of grammatical vulnerability, such as agreement marking, as is evident in documented cases where a child can score within normative range and yet demonstrate clinically significant problems (Schuele & Rice, in preparation). For this reason alone it is essential that the morphemes or structures likely to be vulnerable in SLI grammars be identified and incorporated into assessment batteries. A further reason becomes apparent when we consider the possibility that there may be an inherited component to SLI. In order to evaluate this possibility, accurate ways must be available to identify affected individuals. Morphosyntax is a promising area to search for a possible grammatical phenotype (cf. Tomblin & Buckwalter, chap. 2, and Crago & Gopnik, chap. 3, this volume).

Assessment

The preceding remarks highlight the use of assessment to diagnose the existence of SLI. Another function is to identify possible treatment goals and to evaluate progress in intervention. For these purposes, it is essential that the particulars of the grammar be described, and that it be understood how various surface structures may be linked in underlying representations. For example, plural -*s* can be thought of as a matter of matching real-world information about numbers of things to the word ending. In this case, one would look for a child's ability to say "balls" and not "ball" when shown a picture of three balls. However, if plurals are thought of as also involving agreement relations, then one would want to know if the child could mark NUM in several kinds of linguistic frames, such as "this ball" and "two balls." It could prove to be important to evaluate number marking in the *determiner* + *noun* contexts separately from the *quantifier* + *noun* contexts. It may be premature to conclude, for example, that treatment is complete (or needed) if only the first, but not the second, context is examined. (It is, of course, vitally important to determine a child's ability to produce the final sibilants to rule out possible phonological problems that can contribute to what may appear to be a morphological problem.)

Treatment

A necessary part of intervention planning is to identify appropriate therapy goals. Among the dimensions to be considered are phonology, lexical acquisition, social uses of language, and morphosyntax. It would be a mistake, from the viewpoint developed here, to regard grammatical morphemes as a small part of the grammar that can be easily ignored. Instead, the little functors of the grammar act as essential linguistic operators that serve a central function in the grammar. It may well turn out to be the case that other surface symptomatology is to some extent secondary to these little operators. For example, morphology can serve as valuable cues to lexical acquisition (cf. Rice et al., 1993). A second example is that children unable to demonstrate grammatical flexibility also have fewer resources with which to carry out the fine-tunings necessary for successful discourse with their peers. Thus, grammatical development may be an essential concomitant for the development of the lexicon and social uses of language.

Another important clinical decision is the determination of the order in which to treat linguistic problems. Extrapolating again from the plurals and agreement marking discussed above, if a clinician wishes to target the omission of final -*s* plurals and agreement, the findings suggest that plurals are the target more likely to yield to intervention than is agreement marking. Working with a similar logic, if a child demonstrates limited verbal agreement, according to the Optional Infinitive account, it is likely that he or she will also demonstrate problems with the marking of regular past tense, and that the most appropriate way to approach remediation of the missing agreement is to work first on the tense marking.

Although there is certainly a nontrivial amount of speculation involved in such clinical projections, it is also clear that the study of the morphosyntax of children with SLI does have considerable potential clinical value, ranging from a better understanding of the nature of the underlying problems, to predicted etiological factors, to the details of what to assess and how to plan intervention. Clinicians should not expect the full story to be available immediately, because such investigations require years of effort. There is encouragement to be found, however, in recent advances, many of which are reported in this volume.

REFERENCES

Bishop, D.V.M. (1992). Biological basis of specific language impairment. In P. Fletcher & D. Hall (Eds.), *Specific speech and language disorders in children: Correlates, characteristics, and outcomes* (pp. 2–17). San Diego, CA: Singular Publishing Group.

Chomsky, N. (1992). A minimalist program for linguistic theory. *MIT Occasional Papers in Linguistics, 1*.

Clahsen, H. (1989). The grammatical characterization of developmental dysphasia. *Linguistics, 27,* 897–920.

Clahsen, H. (1992). Linguistic perspectives on specific language impairment. In *Theorie Des Lexikons, Arbeiten Des Sonderforschungsbereichs* 282, Nr. 37. Universitat Dusseldorf.

Curtiss, S., Katz, W., & Tallal, P. (1992). Delay vs. deviance in the language acquisition of language impaired children. *Journal of Speech and Hearing Research, 35,* 373–383.

Gertner, B., Hadley, P.A., & Rice, M.L. (1993, March). *Implications of language limitations for social acceptance in preschool.* Poster presentation at the biennial meeting of the Society for Research in Child Development, New Orleans, LA.

Gopnik, M. (1990). Feature-blindness: A case study. *Language Acquisition, 1,* 139–164.

Gopnik, M., & Crago, M.B. (1991). Familial aggregation of a developmental language disorder. *Cognition, 39,* 1–50.

Hadley, P.A. (1993). *A longitudinal investigation of the auxiliary system in children with specific language impairment.* Unpublished doctoral dissertation, Child Language Program, University of Kansas, Lawrence, KS.

Hadley, P.A., & Rice, M.L. (1991). Conversational responsiveness of speech and language impaired preschoolers. *Journal of Speech and Hearing Research, 34,* 1308–1317.

Haegemann, L. (1991). *Introduction to government and binding theory.* Oxford: Blackwell.

Johnston, J.R. (1988). Specific language disorders in the child. In L. Lass, L. Mc-Reynolds, J. Northern, & D. Yoder (Eds.), *Handbook of speech-language pathology and audiology* (pp. 685–715). Toronto: Decker.

Lahey, M., Liebergott, J., Chesnick, M., Menyuk, P., & Adams, J. (1992). Variability in children's use of grammatical morphemes. *Applied Psycholinguistics, 13,* 373–398.

Leonard, L.B. (1989). Language learnability and specific language impairment in children. *Applied Psycholinguistics, 10,* 179–202.

Leonard, L.B., Bortolini, U., Caselli, M.C., McGregor, K.K., & Sabbadini, L. (1992). Morphological deficits in children with specific language impairment: The status of features in the underlying grammar. *Language Acquisition, 2,* 151–179.

Loeb, D., & Leonard, L. (1991). Subject case marking and verb morphology in normally developing and specifically language-impaired children. *Journal of Speech and Hearing Research, 34,* 340–346.

Oetting, J.B., & Rice, M.L. (1993). Plural acquisition in children with specific language impairments. *Journal of Speech and Hearing Research, 36,* 1236–1248.

Radford, A. (1990). *Syntactic theory and the acquisition of English syntax.* Oxford: Blackwell.

Rice, M.L. (1991). Children with specific language impairment: Toward a model of teachability. In N.A. Krasnegor, D.M. Rumbaugh, R.L. Schiefelbusch, & M. Studdert-Kennedy (Eds.), *Biological and behavioral determinants of language development* (pp. 447–480). Hillsdale, NJ: Lawrence Erlbaum Associates.

Rice, M.L. (1993a). "Don't talk to him: He's weird": The role of language in early social interactions. In A.P. Kaiser & D.B. Gray (Eds.), *Enhancing children's communication: Research foundations for intervention* (pp. 139–158). Baltimore: Paul H. Brookes Publishing Co.

Rice, M.L. (1993b). Social consequences of specific language impairment. In H. Grimm & H. Skowronek (Eds.), *Language acquisition problems and reading disorders: Aspects of diagnosis and intervention* (pp. 111–128). New York: Walter de-Gruyter.

Rice, M.L., & Bode, J.V. (1993). GAPS in the verb lexicons of children with specific language impairment. *First Language, 13,* 113–131.

Rice, M.L., Buhr, J.C., & Nemeth, M.J. (1990). Fast mapping word learning abilities of language delayed preschoolers. *Journal of Speech and Hearing Disorders, 55,* 33–42.

Rice, M.L., Buhr, J., & Oetting, J. (1992). Specific-learning-impaired children's quick incidental learning of words: The effect of a pause. *Journal of Speech and Hearing Research, 35,* 1040–1048.

Rice, M.L., Cleave, P.L., Oetting, J.B., & Pae, S. (1993, March). *Preschoolers' use of syntactic cues in assignment of novel names to unfamiliar mass/count objects.* Poster presentation at the biennial meeting of the Society of Research in Child Development, New Orleans, LA.

Rice, M.L., Hadley, P.A., & Alexander, A.L. (in press). Social biases toward children with speech and language impairments: A correlative causal model of language limitations. *Applied Psycholinguistics, 14.*

Rice, M.L., & Oetting, J.B. (1993). Morphological deficits of children with SLI: Evaluation of number marking and agreement. *Journal of Speech and Hearing Research, 36,* 1249–1257.

Rice, M.L., Oetting, J.B., Marquis, J., Bode, J., & Pae, S. (in press). Frequency of input effects on word comprehension of children with specific language impairment. *Journal of Speech and Hearing Research.*

Rice, M.L., Sell, M.A., & Hadley, P.A. (1991). Social interactions of speech and language impaired children. *Journal of Speech and Hearing Research, 34,* 1299–1307.

Rice, M.L., & Wexler, K. (1993, July). *Clause structure and inflection in SLI: Preliminary observations and predictions.* Paper presented at the Sixth International Congress for the Study of Child Language, Trieste, Italy.

Schuele, C.M., & Rice, M.L. (in preparation). *Language disordered? Diagnostic limitations of standardized language assessment.*

Tallal, P., & Piercy, M. (1973). Defects of nonverbal auditory perception in children with developmental aphasia. *Nature, 241,* 468–469.

Wexler, K. (1992, November). *Optional infinitives, head movement, and the economy of derivations in child grammar.* Occasional Paper #45, Center for Cognitive Science, MIT.

6

Some Problems Facing Accounts of Morphological Deficits in Children with Specific Language Impairments

Laurence B. Leonard

IN RECENT YEARS, THE TERM *specific language impairment* (SLI) has been applied to a collection of characteristics seen in certain children with language-learning problems. These characteristics are: 1) a significant deficit in language ability, 2) normal hearing, 3) age-appropriate scores on tests of nonverbal intelligence, 4) no signs of frank neurological impairment, and 5) no symptoms of impaired reciprocal social| interaction| suggestive of autism. Children sharing these attributes do not constitute a homogeneous group. For example, they differ in the severity of their language deficits and in the degree to which problems of language comprehension accompany problems of language production. However, despite several worthy attempts, it has been difficult to arrive at meaningful and empirically reliable subcategories for these children. Consequently, researchers often place children with SLI into a single subject group.

A number of investigators have attempted to uncover the factors that contribute to SLI (see Bishop, 1992; Johnston, 1988; Rice, 1991, for recent reviews). Among the more important findings are those documenting familial concentration of SLI (e.g., Tallal, Ross, & Curtiss, 1989; Tomblin, 1989; Tomblin & Buckwalter, chap. 2, this volume). However, the field is far from having a comprehensive theory of this problem. More recently, several different research groups have set their sights on the more modest goal of accounting for one of the common profiles seen in children with SLI: a mild-to-moderate deficit in a range of language areas and a more serious deficit in the area of grammatical morphology (e.g., Clahsen, 1989; Gopnik, 1990; Leonard, 1989; 1992; Rice & Oetting, 1991). Unfortunately, although these

---

The work reported here was funded by NIDCD research grant DC00458.

accounts have contributed valuable information, each is incomplete, even for this narrower aspect of SLI.

This chapter discusses some of the obstacles to development of a complete account of the morphological limitations in children with SLI. Three types of problems are identified, and some possible solutions are proposed. To provide a context for these problems, let us begin with a brief review of some current accounts of the morphological difficulties in these children.

TWO TYPES OF ACCOUNTS OF MORPHOLOGICAL DEFICITS IN CHILDREN WITH SLI

The diverse accounts of the extraordinary morphological difficulties seen in children with SLI can be placed into two broad theoretic categories. First are the accounts that assume processing limitations on the part of children with SLI. Accounts falling in the second category are those that assume a fundamental deficit in the underlying grammars of these children. An example of each type is presented here.

Processing Limitations: An Example

One example of a processing account can be labeled the *surface* hypothesis. According to this account, children with SLI experience extraordinary difficulty in the area of morphology because many grammatical morphemes in English take the form of word-final nonsyllabic consonants and unstressed syllables that do not appear in positions (namely, clause-final position) in which significant lengthening occurs. Such morphemes have shorter durations than adjacent morphemes; hence, they may be more difficult to perceive. Because they are subject to final consonant deletion and weak syllable deletion, they are also challenging in production.

It is assumed that children with SLI are marginally capable of perceiving and producing final consonants and weak syllables, but that they have a limited processing capacity that is severely taxed when such challenging forms play a morphological role. That is, when forms such as final consonants and weak syllables are separate morphemes, the child must perform additional operations, such as discovering the grammatical functions of the forms and placing the forms in (or retrieving them from) the proper cell of a morphological paradigm. It is assumed that these additional operations render the already difficult forms vulnerable to loss (Leonard, 1989, 1992). In other respects, the manner in which children with SLI build morphological paradigms is assumed to resemble that of nonaffected children. For example, it is assumed that those grammatical functions that have clear semantic correlates will be hypothesized before those that do not.

Together these assumptions suggest that, for example, [s] will appear earlier (and be used more frequently) in a word such as *box* than in a plural noun form such as *rocks,* and that it will appear earlier (and be used more frequently) in *rocks* than in a third person singular verb form such as *knocks.* In the first instance, [s] is part of the lexical item *box* and requires no additional operations. In *rocks,* however, [s] must be extracted from the stem and placed in the plural cell of a paradigm, in the case of perception, or retrieved from the plural cell of a paradigm and combined with the stem, in the case of production. Similar operations are also involved for the [s] in the verb form *knocks.* However, because the semantic correlates for verb agreement are less clear than those for noun plural, the grammatical function of this form is hypothesized later.

Deficits in the Underlying Grammar: An Example

One of the accounts in which the underlying grammars of children with SLI are assumed to be awry can be traced to the work of Clahsen (1989). In an investigation of German-speaking children with SLI, Clahsen concluded that the underlying grammars of these children did not permit agreement relations among sentence constituents. Specifically, the children had difficulty with determiners that must agree with the noun, finite verbs, auxiliaries, and copula forms that must agree with the subject, and case markings whose particular case assignment is controlled by the verb. However, the children showed no particular difficulty with participle inflections, which do not involve agreement. (Hereafter, this account is termed the *agreement deficit* hypothesis.)

Rice and Oetting (1993) and Rice (chap. 5, this volume) have offered a variant of the agreement deficit hypothesis based on data obtained from a large group of English-speaking children with SLI. These investigators observed that the children with SLI produced both the noun plural -*s* and the third person singular verb inflection -*s* with lower percentages in obligatory contexts than did a group of younger, nonaffected children matched for mean length of utterance (MLU). Nevertheless, the percentages for noun plural were quite high for the children with SLI, and instances of overregularizations were observed (e.g., **fishes, *mans*). These findings prompted Rice and Oetting to propose that the group differences for the third person singular verb inflection reflected a more fundamental problem in the children with SLI.

In the linguistic framework adopted by Rice and Oetting (1991), the number marking of the plural noun involves agreement because determiners (e.g., *a, some, this, these*) must agree with the noun in number. However, this agreement seems to differ in kind from the agreement in which the third person singular verb inflection is involved. In the latter, the subject is in specifier position and the verb is in head position, whereas, in the former, both the determiner and the noun are in head positions (see Rice, chap. 5, this volume).

According to Rice and Oetting, the grammars of children with SLI lack the structure necessary for specifier–head agreement in particular, not agreement in general. However, this is not to say that the problem is narrow in scope. Specifier–head agreement is required at many points in the grammar. For example, subject case is assigned through this type of agreement. Therefore, this proposal covers errors such as *her* for *she,* as well as omissions of verb inflections, auxiliaries, and copula forms.

THREE OBSTACLES TO ACCOUNTS OF MORPHOLOGICAL DIFFICULTIES IN CHILDREN WITH SLI

The three problems described here are discussed within the context of the surface and agreement deficit hypotheses. However, it should be kept in mind that each problem poses a challenge to processing accounts in general, all accounts that assume deficits in the underlying grammar, or both.

Language Specificity

The version of the agreement deficit hypothesis advanced by Rice and Oetting (1993) differs from that of Clahsen (1989) in that it proposes that only certain types of agreement are lacking in children with SLI. The rationale for this position is that the children with SLI studied by Rice and Oetting showed productive use of noun plurals, which seem to involve head–head agreement. However, as noted above, Clahsen found that the children he studied had problems with determiner–noun agreement, as well as with other types of agreement. The solution to this seeming discrepancy is that determiner–noun agreement in German must involve specifier–head agreement rather than head–head agreement. Indeed, linguistic analyses of the two languages may find compelling evidence for assuming that the grammars of English and German are configured differently with regard to the determiner–noun relationship.

Unfortunately, this is but one example where results from children with SLI in one language seem to be different from those in another language. Two other examples can be seen in Tables 1 and 2.

The data in Table 1 come from a recent study of Italian-speaking children with SLI reported by Leonard, Bortolini, Caselli, McGregor, and Sabbadini (1992). The children ranged in age from 4;0 (years; months) to 6;0 and in mean length of utterance (MLU) in words from 1.9 to 4.3. Among the grammatical morpheme types examined were three pertinent to the discussion here: articles (one type of determiner), noun plural inflections, and third person singular verb inflections. Italian articles not only mark definiteness; they must also agree with the noun in number and gender. Noun plural inflections are

Table 1. Mean percentages of use of grammatical morphemes in obligatory contexts by Italian-speaking children with specific language impairment (ISLI) and Italian-speaking children without SLI matched for mean length of utterance (IND-MLU) studied by Leonard, Bortolini, Caselli, McGregor, and Sabbadini (1992)

Grammatical morpheme	ISLI (%)	IND-MLU (%)
Articles	41	83
Noun plural	87	89
Third person singular verb	93	93

marked for gender as well as number. The Italian third person singular verb inflection functions in a manner similar to its English equivalent (although it can be applied to certain contexts in which English employs the present progressive). However, unlike the case for English, there is an inflection for each person and number in Italian.

These children's percentages of use in obligatory contexts of each of these grammatical morpheme types were compared to those computed for a group of younger Italian-speaking children without SLI (age 2;6–3;6) matched according to MLU. The Italian-speaking children with SLI were found to be significantly more limited than the control children in their use of articles. The two groups were comparable in their (considerable) use of noun plural and third person singular verb inflections.

For these data to fit the agreement deficit hypothesis, it must be assumed that the underlying grammar of Italian is configured in a way that differs from both German and English. To account for the difficulty with articles shown by the children with SLI, it must be assumed that the determiner–noun relationship involves specifier–head agreement. However, noun plural inflections were not especially difficult, suggesting that these inflections do not enter into agreement with determiners in Italian. Complicating all of this is the observation that third person singular verb inflections were not problematic for these children, yet in both German and English, inflections of this type are assumed to involve specifier–head agreement.

Table 2 is a summary of some relevant data obtained from Hebrew-speaking children with SLI reported in Rom and Leonard (1990). These children ranged in age from 4;4 to 5;3 and in MLU in words from 1.8 to 3.4. The control children were matched according to MLU; they ranged in age from 2;4 to 3;3.

Unlike English and Italian, Hebrew does not employ articles. Instead it uses a noun prefix to mark definiteness. This form does not change with number or gender. There is no marker for the indefinite. As in Italian, noun plurals mark gender as well as number. Present verb inflections in Hebrew

Table 2. Mean percentages of use of grammatical morphemes in obligatory contexts by Hebrew-speaking children with specific language impairment (HSLI) and Hebrew-speaking children without SLI matched for mean length of utterance (HND-MLU) studied by Rom and Leonard (1990)

Grammatical morpheme	HSLI (%)	HND-MLU (%)
Definite prefix	84	95
Noun plural	100	100
Present inflections	94	97

agree with the subject in number and gender. Person is not distinguished in the present tense.

A comparison of the percentages of use in obligatory contexts between the children with SLI and the control group revealed a difference only for the definite prefix. However, even this grammatical morpheme type was used to a considerable degree by the children with SLI. According to Clahsen (1989), definiteness is an inherent feature of articles that does not depend upon agreement. Thus, for this morpheme type, assumptions about the configuration of Hebrew grammar are not crucial. For noun plurals and present verb inflections, however, the problems return. Specifically, we must assume that noun plurals involve head–head agreement as in English, but that present verb inflections do not involve the specifier–head agreement that is assumed for English.

It is highly likely that languages with such distinct typologies as English, German, Hebrew, and Italian have underlying grammars that are configured differently. In fact, the explication of some of these differences has been a goal of recent research in child language (e.g., Hyams, 1992). The problem is that until proposed distinctions are agreed upon, any attempts to attribute cross-linguistic differences in the morphology of children with SLI to differences in the configuration of the languages' underlying grammars will be speculative, at best.

Some of the processing accounts seem less vulnerable to the types of language specificity problems described here, principally because they do not rely on such fine-grained assumptions about grammatical structure. However, in their present form they are not well equipped to handle certain types of cross-linguistic differences.

For example, because the surface hypothesis places importance on the duration of grammatical morphemes, free-standing syllabic morphemes, such as articles, should be less problematic for children with SLI who are acquiring French than for similar children acquiring English and Italian. This is because in French the durations of unstressed syllables (such as articles) and stressed syllables are more similar than in these other languages. In French, stressed syllables are approximately one and one-half times longer than unstressed syllables, whereas in English and Italian, stressed syllables are often more than two times longer than unstressed syllables (Fant, Kruckenberg, & Nord, 1991; Farnetani & Vayra, 1991). This similarity between stressed and unstressed syllables contributes to the perception that all non–clause-final syllables in French have approximately equal stress (e.g., Ladefoged, 1975).

However, the differences in the metrical patterns of these languages might also play a role. As noted by Gerken (1991), English-speaking children's use of articles is made difficult, not only because these morphemes are unstressed, but also because they frequently enter into an iambic (weak syllable–strong syllable) pattern with a following stressed syllable (e.g., *a ball, the car*). Such a pattern runs counter to the dominant trochaic (strong syllable–weak syllable) pattern of multisyllabic English words. French, however, has a dominant iambic pattern. For children acquiring this language, then, the acquisition of articles is a matter of acquiring new morphemes, but not a new metrical pattern in which they are to be used. Consequently, it is quite likely that French-speaking children with SLI would show greater use of articles than children with SLI who are acquiring other languages; however, this advantage could be as much due to the metrical patterns of the respective languages as to the relative duration of the articles.

Low Percentages with Productivity

Too often researchers are divided into those who place emphasis on such measures as percentage of use in obligatory contexts and those who are interested in questions of productivity and contrastivity. Investigators such as Gopnik (1990) and Crago and Gopnik (chap. 3, this volume) correctly note that percentages of use in obligatory contexts say very little about the child's underlying grammar. For example, a child might produce noun plurals only in appropriate contexts (never in inappropriate contexts as in *one cars*), and show evidence of productivity in the form of overregularizations such as *sheeps*. Such achievements, however, are not reflected in the percentage of use in obligatory contexts.

However, percentages of use provide valuable data in their own right, a fact often missed by researchers steeped in the methodological traditions of linguistics. The noun plural data presented by Rice (chap. 5, this volume) serve as one example. Children with SLI showed lower percentages of use of this grammatical morpheme than did children without SLI matched for MLU. However, percentages were quite high and evidence of productivity was found. Linguists might regard a finding of this type as reflecting only a performance limitation, but if such limitations are consistent, they constitute the problem to explain.

Performance limitations can be more dramatic than those seen in Rice's data. An example is shown in Table 3. The data reported in this table come from a group of English-speaking children with SLI and their MLU-matched controls who participated in the investigation reported by Leonard et al. (1992). The children with SLI ranged in age from 3;8 to 5;7 and in MLU in words from 2.7 to 4.2. The MLU controls ranged in age from 2;11 to 3;4.

The children with SLI showed significantly lower percentages of use of the regular past inflection -ed in obligatory contexts than the MLU-matched controls. Some of these percentages were quite low. Nevertheless, seven of the children produced overregularizations such as *throwed.

How can we account for this dual finding of lower percentages than expected, along with productivity in the form of overregularization? One approach to this problem might be found through an adaptation of the learnability framework of Pinker (1984). In this framework, inflections are assumed to be stored in lexical entries as sets of equations, such as *tense = present* and *subjects' number = plural*. To account for how appropriate equations are learned, Pinker proposes that children create paradigms. These are matrix representations containing cells formed by a conjunction of levels of different dimensions. For example, a paradigm might contain the dimensions of *number* and *gender* with the levels of singular and plural, and masculine and feminine, respectively.

In Pinker's (1984) framework, children initially create word-specific paradigms. These paradigms remain in the grammar. In fact, for each word the child learns thereafter, a new word-specific paradigm is created. Of

Table 3.   Percentage of use in obligatory contexts of regular past inflection and presence (+) or absence (−) of overregularization by English-speaking children with specific language impairment (ESLI) and English-speaking children without SLI matched for mean length of utterance (END-MLU) studied by Leonard et al. (1992)

ESLI			END-MLU		
Child	Percentage	Overregularization	Child	Percentage	Overregularization
1	14	−	1	50	−
2	0	−	2	75	−
3	16	−	3	33	−
4	60	+	4	71	+
5	40	+	5	52	+
6	9	+	6	71	+
7	72	+	7	28	−
8	29	+	8	93	−
9	12	+	9	85	+
10	71	+	10	90	+
M	32			65	

course, at some point, children's inflectional systems become productive. For example, hearing some word in its present form, the child can produce the appropriate past tense form. This becomes possible because the word-specific paradigms contribute to the development of general paradigms. A general paradigm is a matrix containing the inflections free of stems. General paradigms then apply to partially filled, word-specific paradigms to fill out the rest of their cells. Importantly, both word-specific and general paradigms can vary in strength as a function of the frequency of the input and competition from candidate rules. (This property of Pinker's [1984] framework is easy to overlook because his is a symbol-processing theory rather than a connectionist model. On close inspection, differences between these two types of frameworks are less marked in the early phases of morphological learning. For example, in Pinker's theory, attested pairs such as *throw–threw, blow–blew,* and *know–knew* could, in principle, serve as the basis of a general paradigm, in other words, a regular rule. However, the appearance of *glow–glowed, sew–sewed, row–rowed,* and the like, with the more applicable inflection *-ed,* which applies as well to stems of many other phonetic shapes, will serve to confine the [o]–[u] pair to particular word-specific paradigms. But this process is not instantaneous; only when *-ed* becomes established does this form become impervious to the effects of input frequency and alternative rules.)

To apply this framework to the problem of low percentages of use with productivity, let us assume that a child notes from the ambient language forms such as *jump* in a present context but *jumped* in a past context, *walk* in a present context but *walked* in a past context, and *laugh* in a present context but *laughed* in a past context. The child also hears *put* in a present and a past context. For still other verbs, such as *talk* and *drink,* the child only hears the forms used in a present context.

According to the Pinker framework, the child forms word-specific paradigms of the form seen in (1) (a)–(f):

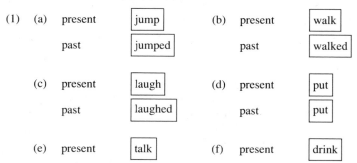

From word-specific paradigms such as these, the child abstracts the common material and forms a general paradigm as in (2):

(2)   present

        past   -ed

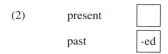

The general paradigm then serves as the basis for splitting as yet undivided word-specific paradigms, and filling in any missing cells in these paradigms. This can be seen in (3) (a)–(b):

(3) (a)   present   talk   (b)   present   drink

           past   talked   past   drinked

As the child encounters additional instances of *talked* in past contexts, the strength of this particular word-specific paradigm is increased directly and this, in turn, feeds back to the general paradigm, strengthening the latter as well. At some point, the child will also encounter *drank* and this form will compete with **drinked*. The overregularization will not be replaced immediately. However, with additional encounters, the irregular form *drank* will replace **drinked* in the paradigm.

According to processing accounts such as the surface hypothesis, children with SLI acquire word-specific and general paradigms in the same manner as children without SLI, but their limited processing capacity makes inflections with difficult surface characteristics more vulnerable to loss when combined with the operations of paradigm building. Consequently, a greater number of encounters with these inflections will be needed before the same number of word-specific paradigms are acquired, with the same strength. However, once this number of word-specific paradigms is, in fact, achieved with sufficient strength, general paradigms will result.

This set of assumptions is highly testable. Specifically, at the point at which overregularizations first occur, the MLUs of children with SLI should be higher than those of children without SLI, but the percentages of use in obligatory contexts should be the same in the two groups of children.

Given this account, the problem of low percentages of use with productivity translates into the question of why, once a general paradigm is formed, the remaining word-specific paradigms fill so slowly with the correct forms. One plausible answer is that unsuccessful applications of the paradigm operations (which are expected to be more frequent in these children because of the assumed capacity limitations) result in the placement of an incomplete entry, namely, the bare stem, in the cell requiring the inflected form. The product of such unsuccessful applications will resemble the case in which the past and present forms are identical, as in (1) (d) above. Because the cell for past is filled, successful applications of the operation will result in competition between the correctly inflected form and the bare stem. To expunge the bare stem, a greater number of encounters (indeed, correctly processed encounters) will be needed than would be the case if the cell had been empty at the outset. Similarly, once a general paradigm is formed, insertion of the correct inflection into the cell for these particular words will meet with greater resistance, hence, will require more time.

This interpretation could represent a possible solution to the problem of accounting for the lower percentages of use seen in children with SLI, even when these children show evidence of productivity. (One detail not explained by this solution is the observation that two of the seven children with SLI who exhibited overregularizations also used -ed with an irregular past form. In each case, this was *broked. However, these two children—subjects 4 and 7 in Table 3—showed percentages of use in obligatory contexts that were as high as those of the children without SLI who produced overregularizations. Therefore, it is not clear that double markings of this type are to be found in the speech of children with SLI who at once show low percentages and overregularizations.) One way to assess the merits of this proposal would be to conduct a teaching experiment with these children. Specifically, we might attempt to teach them to use regular past inflections in novel words, as well as in words already in their lexicons in bare stem form. If this proposal is correct, the children should show more rapid use of the inflection with the new words than with the familiar words because the past tense cells for the new words should not already be filled with inappropriate forms.

There is an alternative solution to the problem of low percentages of use with productivity in children with SLI. Marcus et al. (1992) have proposed that when young children without SLI overregularize, the irregular past forms are located in the word-specific paradigms, but the children fail to retrieve them. Such retrieval problems can be expected with some (small) probability because of the weaker memory traces in young children as a result of more limited exposure to the words. Because a past form is, nonetheless, required in the situation, the regular -ed, which is available from the general paradigm, is affixed to the stem.

An assumption of retrieval failure seems highly applicable to the case of children with SLI. Relative to age-matched controls, children with SLI have been found to recall fewer words on memory tasks, and to produce the names of objects and actions less accurately and more slowly on naming tasks (Kail & Leonard, 1986). It would seem reasonable to expect, therefore, that these children would also be less successful in their retrieval of irregular past forms.

Unfortunately, this alternative solution is incomplete because it is silent on the matter of how the regular inflection -ed can be so readily applied in instances of failed retrieval when it is used with relatively low percentages in obligatory contexts. This shortcoming renders the first of these alternative solutions more satisfactory.

The Nature of Limited Processing Capacity

For accounts such as the surface hypothesis to be maximally useful, they must provide greater detail regarding the notion of limited processing capacity. As Johnston (chap. 7, this volume) has pointed out, this notion carries the advantage of being applicable to a broad range of performance data. Unfortunately, as she also noted, this breadth pays a price in precision. It is simply not yet clear just which types of operations place the greatest demands on processing capacity, or how these operations interact with one another.

However, it seems that this question can be approached, at least with regard to the specific assumptions of the surface hypothesis. A chief assumption of this hypothesis is that the processing capacity limitations of children with SLI are severely taxed when consonants and syllables with challenging surface characteristics are involved in the process of paradigm building. The direction taken thus far in this line of research has been to compare children with SLI who are acquiring languages with challenging grammatical morphemes to children with SLI who are acquiring languages whose grammatical morphemes pose few if any surface problems. However, when only the surface difficulty is manipulated in a systematic manner, the question of processing capacity is not directly tested.

A parallel program of research should control for surface characteristics and manipulate the presumed degree of processing required in the paradigm building process. To illustrate how this might be done, we adopt again the framework of Pinker (1984). According to Pinker's learnability procedures, children build paradigms by searching for common material for one dimension at a time. For example, in building paradigms involving nouns, the child acquiring English might look for common material that pertains to *number;* as a result the plural noun inflection -*s* is learned. However, the task is more complicated for the English verb inflection -*s,* because this form represents the conjunction of *number* and *person* (and, of course, *tense*). Thus, when the child searches for forms pertaining to *number,* -*s* will become a candidate for singular, but it will not be incorporated into the paradigm because other instances of singular verbs will be noted that do not have the -*s* form. That is, the child will note such examples as *I like* and *you* (singular) *like,* as well as *she likes.* For morphemes of this type, the child must simultaneously consider two dimensions (e.g., *number* and *person*) to be successful. Only when *person* is considered along with *number* will -*s* find its rightful place in the paradigm. According to Pinker, greater processing capacity is required to consider two dimensions simultaneously than to consider one dimension at a time.

An ideal examination of the role of processing capacity limitations would be one in which children with SLI acquiring a language with a fusional morphology are compared to similar children who are acquiring a language with an agglutinating morphology. The former type of morphology is seen when each inflection represents a conjunction of dimensions (e.g., distinct forms for first person singular, second person singular, third person singular, first person plural, second person plural, and third person plural). In an agglutinating morphology, in contrast, each inflection represents only one dimension (e.g., there is a form for third person that is distinct from the form for singular).

To see how a comparison involving the distinction between fusional and agglutinating morphology might be useful, assume that the inflections of two different languages are comparable in having challenging surface characteristics, but that the morphology of one is agglutinating and the morphology of the other is fusional, as in the word-specific paradigms in (4) (a) and (b). In each paradigm, the stem is *fov* and each italicized letter in (4) (a) and (b) corresponds to a distinct inflection. According to Pinker (1984), the child in each case looks for common material for one dimension at a time. For example, in (4) (a), the child might hypothesize *number* and discover the common elements y for singular and z for plural. The child might then hypothesize *tense* and identify the common elements m for present and n for past:

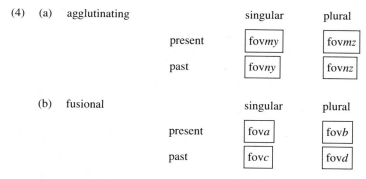

(4) (a) agglutinating

	singular	plural
present	fov*my*	fov*mz*
past	fov*ny*	fov*nz*

(b) fusional

	singular	plural
present	fov*a*	fov*b*
past	fov*c*	fov*d*

For the morphology reflected in (4) (b), the task is not so simple. If the child hypothesizes *number,* he or she will not find any common material. A similar outcome occurs if he or she considers *tense*. Only when the child begins to consider both of these dimensions simultaneously will he or she arrive at the correct paradigm. Because this type of paradigm places greater demands on processing capacity, children with SLI who are acquiring a morphology of this type should show significantly less use of appropriate inflections than children with SLI who are acquiring a morphology such as the one in (4) (a). Of course, these differences would be expected among children without SLI, as well. To support the hypothesis that children with SLI are especially vulnerable to problems when paradigm building requires greater processing capacity, the differences between children with SLI and

MLU-matched controls (favoring the latter) should be greater in the language with fusional morphology than in the language with agglutinating morphology.

Processing capacity limitations could also be examined through a comparison of children with SLI acquiring two different fusional languages that are generally challenging in the surface characteristics of their grammatical morphemes. In one language, each inflection could represent the conjunction of two different dimensions (e.g., *person* and *number*), whereas in the other each inflection could represent the conjunction of three different dimensions (e.g., *person, number,* and *gender*). The latter would be expected to pose greater difficulty because the child must simultaneously consider three, rather than two, dimensions in order to arrive at the correct paradigm.

SUMMARY

A common profile in children with SLI who are acquiring English is a particularly notable weakness in grammatical morphology. There have been several recent attempts to account for this profile. These accounts differ in terms of whether they assume processing capacity limitations but an otherwise intact language-learning mechanism in children with SLI, or whether the underlying grammars of these children are assumed to differ from those of younger children without SLI.

In this chapter three problems facing these accounts are considered. One of these is that findings of cross-linguistic differences among children with SLI seem to be outpacing investigators' ability to predict such differences on the basis of the underlying grammars assumed for these languages. Another problem is that, in emphasizing either low percentages of use in obligatory contexts or questions of productivity, advocates of each type of account have made no attempt to explain the fact that children with SLI can at once exhibit productivity with a grammatical morpheme and lower-than-expected percentages of use of the grammatical morpheme in obligatory contexts. The third problem considered is the as yet unspecified nature of limited processing capacity that certain accounts attribute to children with SLI.

Each of these problems can be solved, and a few ways in which they might be approached are discussed here. These are not the only problems facing accounts of the morphological deficits in children with SLI. However, it seems clear that until they are solved we won't be ready to move to the larger task of determining the precise role that problems of morphology play in specific language impairment.

REFERENCES

Bishop, D.V.M. (1992). The underlying nature of specific language impairment. *Journal of Child Psychology & Psychiatry & Allied Disciplines, 33*(1), 3–66.

Clahsen, H. (1989). The grammatical characterization of developmental dysphasia. *Linguistics, 27,* 897–920.

Fant, G., Kruckenberg, A., & Nord, L. (1991). Durational correlates of stress in Swedish, French, and English. *Journal of Phonetics, 19,* 351–365.

Farnetani, E., & Vayra, M. (1991). Word- and phrase-level aspects of vowel reduction in Italian. *Proceedings of the Twelfth International Congress of Phonetic Sciences* (Vol. 2, 14–17).

Gerken, L. (1991). The metrical basis for children's subjectless sentences. *Journal of Memory and Language, 30,* 431–451.

Gopnik, M. (1990). Feature blindness: A case study. *Language Acquisition, 1,* 139–164.

Hyams, N. (1992). A reanalysis of null subjects in child language. In J. Weissenborn, H. Goodluck, & T. Roeper (Eds.), *Theoretical issues in language acquisition* (pp. 249–267). Hillsdale, NJ: Lawrence Erlbaum Associates.

Johnston, J.R. (1988). Specific language disorders in the child. In N. Lass, L. McReynolds, J. Northern, & D. Yoder (Eds.), *Handbook of speech-language pathology and audiology* (pp. 685–715). Toronto: B.C. Decker.

Kail, R., & Leonard, L. (1986). Word-finding abilities in language-impaired children. *ASHA Monographs, 25.*

Ladefoged, P. (1975). *A course in phonetics.* New York: Harcourt Brace Jovanovich.

Leonard, L.B. (1989). Language learnability and specific language impairment in children. *Applied Psycholinguistics, 10,* 179–202.

Leonard, L. (1992). The use of morphology by children with specific language impairment: Evidence from three languages. In R. Chapman (Ed.), *Processes in language acquisition and disorders* (pp. 186–201). St. Louis, MO: Mosby-Yearbook.

Leonard, L.B., Bortolini, U., Caselli, M.C., McGregor, K.K., & Sabbadini, L. (1992). Morphological deficits in children with specific language impairment: The status of features in the underlying grammar. *Language Acquisition, 2,* 151–179.

Marcus, G., Pinker, S., Ullmann, M., Hollander, M., Rosen, T., & Xu, F. (1992). Overregularization in language acquisition. *Monographs of the Society for Research in Child Development, 57* (4, Serial No. 228).

Pinker, S. (1984). *Language learnability and language development.* Cambridge, MA: Harvard University Press.

Rice, M.L. (1991). Children with specific language impairment: Toward a model of teachability. In N. Krasnegor, D.M. Rumbaugh, R.L. Schiefelbusch, & M. Studdert-Kennedy (Eds.), *Biological and behavioral determinants of language development* (pp. 447–480). Hillsdale, NJ: Lawrence Erlbaum Associates.

Rice, M.L., & Oetting, J.B. (1991, October). *Morphological deficits of SLI children: Evaluation of number marking and agreement.* Paper presented at the Boston University Conference on Language Development, Boston.

Rice, M.L., & Oetting, J.B. (1993). Morphological deficits of children with SLI: Evaluation of number marking and agreement. *Journal of Speech and Hearing Research, 36,* 1249–1257.

Rom, A., & Leonard, L. (1990). Interpreting deficits in grammatical morphology in specifically language-impaired children: Preliminary evidence from Hebrew. *Clinical Linguistics & Phonetics, 4,* 93–105.

Tallal, P., Ross, R., & Curtiss, S. (1989). Familial aggregation in specific language impairment. *Journal of Speech and Hearing Disorders, 54,* 167–173.

Tomblin, J.B. (1989). Familial concentration of developmental language impairment. *Journal of Speech and Hearing Disorders, 54,* 287–295.

7

Cognitive Abilities of Children with Language Impairment

Judith R. Johnston

I BEGAN MY STUDIES OF language disorders as a clinician. Even now, when I think of "specific language impairment," I think of these children:

— Mark, a 4-year-old at the two-word stage, assuming the role of his mother in a complicated pretend/play drama set at the movie theatre
— Lisa, a 6-year-old at the one-word stage, laughing at her own puns
— Alex, a 4-year-old with no expressive speech, showing other children in our preschool how to make vegetable tempura

Children with specific language impairment are, by definition, children for whom the development of language and thought is out of phase. Each of the children above had knowledge and competencies far in advance of those expected judging from their language levels. Each had achieved normal range scores on a nonverbal test of intelligence. Each, at times, radiated a fierce intellectual energy that was undeniable. In short, they were classic examples of children who are intellectually normal, although with language delays. The problem is this: by virtually any account of intellect, such children should not exist.

DEVELOPMENTAL RELATIONSHIPS
BETWEEN COGNITION AND LANGUAGE

To understand this paradox, we must consider the many relationships between language and thought, or, to be more precise, between verbal and nonverbal cognition. Studying patterns of human growth, we quickly discover that the

This chapter is an expanded version of a paper presented at the International Symposium on Specific Speech and Language Disorders in Children, Harrogate, England, May 1991, and subsequently published in P. Fletcher & D. Hall (Eds.), *Specific speech and language disorders in children*. London: Whurr. Copyright © 1992 by the Association For All Speech Impaired Children. Adapted by permission.

development of language and thought are interdependent at all stages of life.

First, consider the relationship between cognition and language that is evident during language learning. The nature of this process is controversial, but I am among those who hold that the "language acquisition device" is nothing more or less than the general information processing capabilities that constitute the mind. From this perspective, children learn the language system by applying their powers of observation, organization, and analysis to the examples of language that they hear. Awesome as these powers may be, cognitive scientists have long argued that the mind functions as a limited capacity system, that is, as a system that can do only so much at once. In complex tasks, this restriction may lead to processing "tradeoffs." For example, most drivers can converse while driving—until the traffic gets heavy. Similar phenomena can be seen in young language learners. Toddlers are more likely to use new inflectional morphemes when expressing familiar semantic relations (Leonard, Steckol, & Schwartz, 1978). Utterances with greater propositional complexity are less likely to include all the underlying constituents (Bloom, Miller, & Hood, 1975). Moreover, young children's syntactic errors increase with syllabic complexity (Panagos & Prelock, 1982). The notion of limited capacity certainly seems applicable to these examples. Other principles of mental function, for example, recency and interruption effects in memory or attentional biases toward novelty, also could be shown to influence language learning and use (Pinker, 1989). The most fundamental relationship between cognition and language, then, is that cognitive mechanisms create and constrain language knowledge.

Different relationships between cognition and language are evident when we examine the periods before and after the language-learning period. Before infants can learn to speak, they must learn to think about means and ends, and to understand the limits imposed by the independence of objects (Bates, Benigni, Bretherton, Camaioni, & Volterra, 1979). These nonverbal, cognitive achievements help prepare toddlers to use words as symbolic tools of communication. Once language is learned, however, the dependencies shift. Language becomes a major mode of mental representation, and crucial to many reasoning tasks. Imagery may suffice when the goal is to rearrange the living room or remember a tune, but other goals require the unique power of words to represent just those aspects of objects and events that are pertinent to the problem. Consider the business manager preparing a work assignment plan, or a teenager choosing between two summer jobs. It is hard to imagine success in such tasks without the use of language. Words provide a powerful and flexible way to create nonexistent events for reflection and organization (Olson, 1975).

Normally, language is a well-integrated part of mental life. We apply the organizing forces of nonverbal intellect to learn language in the first place, and we constantly rely upon linguistic symbols for complex reasoning. Language would seem to be both the product and the tool of cognition. If so, specific language impairment should not exist. If language is late and slow to develop, there should be a cognitive reason. If language symbols are poorly controlled, there should be a cognitive consequence.

STUDIES OF COGNITIVE DEVELOPMENT
IN CHILDREN WITH SPECIFIC LANGUAGE IMPAIRMENT

Symbolic Play

About 12 years ago, I, my students, and other investigators began to look more carefully at the putative *normal* intellect of children with specific language impairment. Let me briefly summarize what we have found. One group of studies examined symbolic play in this population. A study by Terrell, Schwartz, Prelock, and Messick (1984) illustrates this line of research. Fifteen children with language impairment and fifteen without were asked to complete the Symbolic Play Test (Lowe & Costello, 1976) and to engage in spontaneous pretend-play activities. The children were all at the one-word stage and had expressive vocabularies of 25–75 words; the group with language impairment was 1 1/2 years older than the group without, that is, 35 months versus 19 months. Play samples were rated according to such criteria as the number of symbolic acts, the number of play units combining two or more symbolic schemes, and the number of play units that focused on actors other than self. The children with language impairment engaged in more complex and mature play than their language peers, but they fell significantly below age expectations. Similar findings have been reported in at least eight other investigations (Brown, Redmond, Bass, Liebergott, & Swope, 1975; Lovell, Hoyle, & Siddall, 1968; Morehead, 1972; Roth & Clark, 1987; Skarakis & Prutting, 1988; Terrell & Schwartz, 1988; Thal & Bates, 1988; Udwin & Yule, 1983).

At the University of British Columbia, a student of mine, Kathleen Capreol, is now replicating the Terrell et al. (1984) study, with two goals in mind: first, to see whether children with language disorder show the same association between delays in language learning and delays in nonverbal symbolic behavior at different stages of language learning, and second, to investigate the relations between symbolic play and nonsymbolic problem solving. Terrell and others have demonstrated that children with specific language impairment are likely to have deficits in symbolic play. But it is not yet clear whether these play deficits represent some special problem with symbolic function, or whether they are merely part of a broader pattern of intellectual impairment.

Although she ruled out children with profound developmental delays, Capreol did not limit her study to children with specific language impairment.

Six of her subjects, however, fell into this category, and the data from these toddlers present an intriguing picture. Each of the children completed standardized language tests and the Symbolic Play Test (Lowe & Costello, 1976), did a series of block construction problems (J. Stiles, personal communication, September 1991), and contributed samples of spontaneous symbolic play and spontaneous language. From these observations, Capreol developed a 3-point profile: expressive language level, symbolic play level, and manipulative problem-solving level. For the children with language impairment, all the profiles show age-appropriate performance in block constructions, as well as the expected developmental gap between block building and language skills. The key finding concerns the level of symbolic play. For three of the children, symbolic play levels are similar to language levels; for the other three, symbolic play scores are at the level of block building. Neither age nor language comprehension distinguishes the two groups, but the children with stronger play skills have larger vocabularies and more word combinations. This finding is corroborated in a recent longitudinal study of four late talkers whose play scores similarly lagged until their vocabularies reached 50 words (Ellis Weismer, Murray-Branch, & Miller, 1991.)

Given the small sample size, Capreol's results cannot be taken as conclusive. They suggest, however, that some children with specific language impairment do manifest *early* symbolic play deficits despite age-level performance on other tasks requiring constructive intelligence. If we accept the arguments of Shore, Bates, Bretherton, Beeghly, and O'Connell (1990) and Pettito (in press) that language and gesture systems have an initial period of independent development, then the early play deficits may, indeed, indicate a special problem with symbolic functions across mode. However, Capreol's data also suggest that once this early phase has passed, growth in symbolic play is linked to language abilities. I return to this theme later, but now we must look at a second group of studies examining cognitive development in children with language impairment.

Conceptual Development

The second group of studies examining cognitive development has used Piagetian paradigms to access conceptual development in children with specific language impairment (Camarata, Newhoff, & Rugg, 1981, 1985; Johnston & Ramstad, 1983; Kamhi, 1981; Siegel, Lees, Allan, & Bolton, 1981; Snyder, 1978). Kamhi's work can be taken as representative of the others. In his study, a group of 5-year-old children with specific language impairment was compared to two groups without specific language impairment, one matched to the group with impairment by mental age and the other by language level. Each of the children was given six reasoning tasks, ranged across the conceptual domains of space, class, and number. As parts of this battery, the children had to sort geometric shapes that varied in size, color, and shape; arrange small toys in order, according to a visible model; determine the relative quantity of two sets of checkers; and recognize geometric shapes by feel. Each of these tasks has a long research history and provides a reliable picture of the maturity of a child's thought. In this light, Kamhi's findings are particularly telling. In each of the six tasks, the children with language impairment outperformed their language-level peers, but failed to reach the performance level of their mental-age peers. Not many of the individual comparisons were statistically significant, but the likelihood of obtaining this consistent pattern of results by chance alone is virtually nil. Moreover, these results are in general accord with those from other studies, including those that have observed older children (Johnston & Ramstad, 1983), and those that have used strictly nonverbal adaptations of the Piagetian tasks (Siegel et al., 1981).

Summary

There have been other efforts to study cognitive development in children with language impairment, but these two bodies of research will serve to provide an initial answer to our question. (See Bishop, 1992, and Johnston, 1988, for comprehensive reviews.) We have seen how theories of the relationship between cognition and language predict that children with specific language impairment should not exist. The reports of symbolic play and conceptual development indicate that, indeed, they don't—at least not in the classic sense. When we observe children with normal nonverbal IQs and serious language delays, they seem to be lacking the conceptual knowledge, the representational abilities, and the reasoning patterns expected for their age.

NATURE OF THE COGNITIVE DISABILITY

Role of Language in Cognitive Impairment

Should we believe these data? Could they merely be reflections of the language disorder itself? Experimenters can minimize the demands for explicit language use, but that scarcely prevents children from using language as an internal mental tool. Perhaps children with language impairment performed less well than their peers only because they lack facility with such inner speech?

Note that this line of argument implies that some mental calculations welcome verbal representation, even if they don't require it. Nonverbal strategies for such problems might exist in principle, but prove to be clumsy or complex in application—leading to breakdowns in reasoning, or to delayed mastery. Whenever mental strategies lead to simpler solutions than nonverbal strategies, the child with a language impairment would be at a developmental disadvantage. Language would be crucial for solving these problems at a given age or stage, if not absolutely.

My first answer to the skeptic is: Yes. Poor performance on symbolic or conceptual tasks could, indeed, reflect a lack of facility with the inner use of language. From one viewpoint, however, that is not the problem with these data—it is their point. Children with serious language impairment lack an important intellectual tool, thus, they are hindered in their development of concepts and world understanding. Rather than treating this relationship between language skills and cognitive development as an experimental design problem, that is, trying to get the language out of cognition, we might learn more if we explicitly studied it.

One such study was recently conducted by Fazio (1990) at Indiana University. The conceptual domain of *number* is one in which language plays a unique developmental role. From the work of Saxe (1979) and others, it seems that children must learn to count before they can solve quantification problems that have any degree of complexity. Number words are normally acquired quite early as part of counting routines. Children work hard to learn all the proper noises, in the proper order: "1, 2, 3, 4, 6, 7, 8, 10." Then they learn to coordinate the noise-making with pointing to the objects in an array. While this learning is underway, children do not control the quantificational meanings of number terms. Preschoolers who can count to five may, nevertheless, be unable to hand you three blocks. They may conclude that a pile of six coins has fewer than a row of four coins, or they may be unable to answer a "How many?" question, despite being able to count. Toward the end of the preschool years, however, children discover the potential utility of counting routines, and begin to use them as verbal "yardsticks," to measure quantities. This opens the door to much more rigorous and explicit numerical reasoning.

So, what happens to the child who can't learn the noises in the first place? Many children with language impairment have exactly this problem. We may quibble about whether semantically empty counting routines really should be considered as language, but they certainly are more verbal than not. Counting would seem to be a good domain in which to investigate the intellectual costs of a verbal deficit.

Fazio (1990) observed 5-year-olds with language impairment in a series of counting tasks. The children recited the longest rote sequence of numbers they could manage, and then applied these rote counting skills to various sets of toys. As they finished counting each set, the children were asked how many toys it contained. The performance of the children with language impairment was compared to two groups of children without language impairment, one matched for mental age and one for language level. The results offer a revealing picture of cognitive weaknesses and strengths. The children with language impairment had considerable difficulty with the counting routines: on average they could only count as far as 6 before they began omitting, repeating, or incorrectly sequencing the terms. The 5-year-olds without language impairment could count to 22. When the children with language impairment tried to count the toys, they had difficulty with one-to-one correspondences, and their verbal routines deteriorated even further. In fact, in all these aspects of counting, the children with language impairment performed much as did their language peers who were 1½ years younger.

There was also, however, an important difference between these groups. When the 3-year-olds were asked, "How many toys are there?" they tended to recount. The children with language impairment did not. Instead, they would often immediately provide the last number they had reached while counting. They seemed to understand the potential significance of counting, and in this way they demonstrated a certain degree of intellectual maturity. Unfortunately, because they were poor counters, their answers were seldom correct.

The ultimate cognitive costs of delayed counting skills are unknown. But, the Fazio (1990) data may help to explain why children with language impairment have demonstrated conceptual delays of 1–5 years in quantification tasks (Johnston & Ramstad, 1983; Kamhi, 1981), and why their school progress in math is only two-thirds the normal pace (Schery, 1980). Difficulty with a verbal tool has impeded their numerical problem solving from the earliest years.

A second explicit study of the role of language in cognition was reported recently by Kamhi and his students (Kamhi, Gentry, & Mauer, 1990). In this experiment, school-age children were taught to solve problems of the sort represented by the story about the man who is trying to get his fox, goose, and corn across the river but can only take two of them across at one time. Half of the children received verbal explanations; the other half received the same verbal explanations accompanied by visual demonstrations with toy objects. For the children without language impairment, learning was equally fast with either teaching method. The children with language impairment in contrast learned three times more slowly when they only heard the verbal explanations. In this case, the cognitive costs of a language deficit are dramatic and clear.

To summarize briefly, there is substantial evidence that children with language impairment show intellectual delays in a number of conceptual domains and at a number of ages. Critics of this literature have raised the possibility that the delays merely reflect the language problem itself, rather than any fundamental deficit in knowledge or in reasoning abilities. My first answer to such critics is: Yes. Language is so integral to normal intellectual function, and so crucial to its development, that children who lack it will be hindered in learning virtually everything. My second answer takes a different tack.

Evidence for Nonverbal Deficits

What the skeptic really wants to know is whether there is *any* evidence to indicate that the cognitive deficits of children with language impairment extend to nonverbal functions. Difficulties with rhythm perception (Kracke, 1975), and memory for spatial arrays (Doehring, 1960; Wyke & Asso, 1979) would seem to suggest purely nonverbal impairments. The most convincing data on this point, however, may come from an imagery study conducted by Johnston and Ellis Weismer (1983). We asked children with and without language impairment at 6.5 and 9.5 years of age to judge whether or not two rows of geometric forms were the same. In one-fourth of the items, both arrays were presented in a vertical orientation. In the remaining items, the right-hand array was rotated about its center either 45°, 90°, or 135°. All the children were screened for their understanding of spatial order concepts and were trained with the apparatus, with emphasis on both accuracy and speed. The ultimate variable for group comparison was response time.

An important feature of this paradigm is that patterns of response across the items can reveal the nature of the mental strategy used to solve the problem (Kosslyn, 1980). If the viewer solves the problem by creating and manipulating mental images, response time proves to be a direct function of the degree of rotation. Extended rotations require more time. If the viewer solves the problem by using verbal symbols to represent the two arrays, the relationship between response time and degree of rotation does not hold. This fact about the task paradigm makes the results of our study particularly interesting. First, data patterns clearly showed that the children with language impairment were using nonverbal, imagistic strategies. Second, although the children with language impairment were accurate in their judgments of order, their response times were substantially slower than those of the control group. This difference remained true even after we adjusted response times to control for any speed differences evident during training. Faced with changing arrays, children with language impairment took longer to make judgments of spatial order. Taken together, these findings indicate that the cognitive deficits of children with language impairment *do* extend to nonverbal functions.

Inadequacy of Current Proposals

There remains little room for doubt on the original question. Across a range of tasks and ages, children with specific language impairment have shown a marked level of intellectual delay. A portion of this disability must reflect the role of language in higher level problem solving. Without normal verbal facility, the child with language impairment is unlikely to reach age-level achievement on tasks that require complex calculations or the consideration of multiple hypothetical states. Another portion of the cognitive disability is nonverbal and can be presumed to be responsible for inefficient learning in many domains, including language. Here many questions remain, especially concerning the fundamental nature of the problem. Some investigators have proposed that children with language impairment have difficulty with such mental activities as hierarchical planning (Cromer, 1983), symbolic function (Morehead, 1972), or hypothesis testing (Nelson, Kamhi, & Apel, 1987). Others have proposed difficulty with basic mechanisms of auditory perception (Ceci, 1983, Eisenson, 1968; Mackworth, Grandstaff, & Pribram, 1973) or short-term memory (Kirchner & Klatzky, 1985). Ultimately, none of these proposals quite fits the data.

Illustrative Data and Interpretation: Capacity Limitations

One of my own studies, with its explanatory arguments, will serve to illustrate the troubled state of current theorizing. Johnston and Smith (1988) observed preschoolers with and without language impairment as they solved a series of complex communication problems. On each item, the children were shown three objects varying systematically in size, color, and identity. In the dimensional sets, two of the objects were similar on the target dimension, for example color, but differed on the second dimension, for example size; the third object differed from the first two in the target dimension, but resembled one of them on the second dimension. For example, one object set might consist of a large green peg, a small green peg, and a large purple peg. In the identity sets, two of the objects were identical, whereas the third differed from the first two in every respect. As each item began, the examiner would point to two similar objects from the set of three. The child's task was to describe these objects to a puppet, so the puppet would know which ones to take.

All the children were successful in the referential task, providing communicatively adequate descriptions. However, the children with language impairment used descriptive strategies that were characteristically different than those provided by their peers. Across all items, responses fell into six categories, illustrated here for an item in which two green pegs are the designated referents.

1. *Deictic*   "This one and that one"
2. *Exhaustive*   "A green big one and a green little one"
3. *Exclusive*   "Not the purple one"
4. *Iterative*   "The green one and the green one"
5. *Partitive*   "Looks like little and green big"
6. *Quantitative*
   grouping   "Two green ones"

Note that all these strategies, save number 1, require dimensional analysis. Strategy 6 additionally requires that the two targeted objects be considered as a quantified set. The key finding was that children with language impairment used the *Quantitative Grouping* strategy much less often than did their peers without language impairments when describing objects that were similar in size or color. Their explanations seldom contained such phrases as "the two red ones." Performance on the identity items was not so restricted. When they did not need to consider separate physical dimensions, the children with language impairment frequently described objects with such phrases as "the two house." This demonstrated their competence with quantity notions and terms. In their use of strategies 2–5, they also demonstrated knowledge of all the requisite dimensional terms. In short, their problem seemed to stem not from a lack of knowledge schemes but from some inability to make use of these schemes to solve a particular problem. To quote from our original report, "Given a task which welcomed the combined use of two higher-level, complex processing routines, the impaired children used one or the other more often than both. The data, thus, seem to represent the variable performance of thinkers who are operating near the limits of their processing resources" (p. 15).

Critique of Capacity Limitations as an Explanation of Cognitive Disability

How viable is this suggestion that children with language impairment suffer limitations in processing capacity? Like other appeals to basic cognitive mechanisms, this explanation has the advantage of being content-free, thus applicable to diverse mental tasks. It differs in this regard from explanations that focus on particular mental activities such as symbol use or hierarchical structuring. The notion of capacity limitations also applies equally well across perceptual modalities, and to both verbal and nonverbal functions. Thus, it fits the growing body of data that indicates visual, as well as auditory, perceptual disorders (Tallal, 1990), and nonverbal as well as verbally mediated deficits. Finally, the notion of capacity limitations predicts both the observed delays in concept/scheme attainment and the observed failures in concept/scheme deployment. Each mental calculation enhances control of available schemes and brings the opportunity for new discoveries. Processing limitations could easily hamper both sorts of mental growth. In sum, explanations of cognitive deficit based on notions of limitations in processing capacity have particular appeal because they seem to fit the broad range of performance data.

As is frequently the case, the broad scope of this explanation may prove to be its Achilles' heel. Global appeals to capacity limitation are difficult to reconcile with evidence of selective impairment, and such evidence definitely exists. Children with specific language impairments do complete the tasks on nonverbal intelligence scales with normal proficiency. They do perform better on nonverbal tasks than on verbal tasks (Kamhi, 1981; Terrell et al., 1984), and, in the world of language, they do seem to learn words faster than grammatical morphemes (Moore, 1990). Any explanation of cognitive impairment must also account for these instances of selective sparing. Arguments about capacity limitations thus must be accompanied by detailed analyses that show why a processing mechanism flawed in this fashion succeeds better on some tasks than on others.

This may be possible. For example, in a recent study of dimensional reasoning (Johnston & Smith, 1989), Smith and I argue that inferences about size demand more processing resources than inferences about color, because size judgments are inherently ordinal and color judgments are not. Explanations of this sort will be more difficult to construct across varying task paradigms and developmental levels, but without them, arguments about capacity limitations will remain hollow. We could begin the analysis by compiling a list of the task parameters that have seemed to account for differential performance. Siegel et al. (1981) note that the more difficult tasks in their battery required "sequential processing." Kamhi (1981) suggests that his difficult tasks required "anticipatory images." Inhelder (1976) implies that the more difficult tasks are those that cannot be solved with "schemes of actual physical action." Clahsen (1989) concludes that grammatical morphemes are relatively difficult because of the "scope" of the rules that govern them. If we can translate these and other similar ideas into the language of processing complexity, we may be able to explain how a pervasive impairment can lead to selective performance deficits.

Should we succeed in this task, however, we face two further problems with the notion of capacity limitation. The first is that some of the evidence of cognitive deficit in children with language impairment comes from tasks that cannot be construed as complex. The reports of Tallal and her colleagues provide the clearest examples (Tallal & Piercy, 1973; Tallal, Stark, Kallman, & Mellits, 1981). In these experiments, children perform such perceptual discrimination tasks as identifying the order of two tones that are presented with various silent intervals between them. The children with language impairment have extreme difficulty with the shortest intervals, but perform as well as their peers with the longer intervals. These findings clearly imply a processing deficit, but not one obviously related to capacity limitations. Rather, as Tallal (1988, p. 164) concludes, "Children with specific developmental language disorders, as a group, are characterized by an inability to perceive and to produce information rapidly in time." At the very least, it would seem that cognitive processing explanations of intellectual impairment will need to invoke limitations in rate as well as capacity. Or will they?

This question is prompted by the final problem with the notion of capacity limitation. In many recent models of cognition, capacity is treated as a matter of function, not structure (Chi & Gallagher, 1982; Kail & Bisanz, 1982). Thus construed, capacity is tantamount to workload, or accomplishment, within a given unit of time. Work that is more rapid, more efficient, and/or done with more powerful mental schemes, can lead to increased capacity. In contrast, slower rates of processing, less efficient access to information, or the need to use more schemes of narrow scope can lead to capacity limitations. In such a system, "capacity" is the epiphenomenal product of an interaction of variables such as rate, efficiency, and power. Capacity may be the construct we can measure best, and it may be a useful heuristic for intervention planning, but it may not prove to be the best explanation.

RESEARCH ACHIEVEMENTS AND CHALLENGES

The developmental relationships between cognition and language make it unlikely that a child could be seriously delayed in language acquisition and otherwise normal in intellect. Research since the early 1980s has revealed that children with specific language impairment do, in fact, show cognitive delays and deficits across a considerable range of tasks. The task for researchers now is to understand the nature of the disorder that underlies these observations.

In the meantime, clinicians can find both comfort and challenge in our findings. As Peter Farb (1974, p. 367) wrote, "Language so interpenetrates the experience of being human that neither language nor behavior can be understood without knowledge of both." The work of the 1980s has proven that children with specific language impairment do, after all, share in this human experience; therein lies the comfort. We can confidently use our knowledge of the normal relationships between language and thought to inform our intervention practice. But therein, also, lies the challenge. To understand the learning patterns and life experiences of children with language impairment, we must understand both their language and their thought. If we sometimes fall short of this goal, we should neither be surprised nor discouraged, for the scope of our inquiry has become the mind itself.

REFERENCES

Bates, E., Benigni, L., Bretherton, I., Camaioni, L., & Volterra, V. (1979). *The emergence of symbols: Cognition and communication in infancy.* New York: Academic Press.

Bishop, D.V.M. (1992). The underlying nature of specific language impairment. *Journal of Child Psychology & Psychiatry & Allied Disciplines, 33* (1), 3–66.

Bloom, L., Miller, P., & Hood, L. (1975). Variation and reduction as aspects of competence in language development. In A. Pick (Ed.), *Minnesota Symposia on Child Psychology* (Vol. 9, pp. 3–55). Minneapolis: University of Minnesota Press.

Brown, J., Redmond, A., Bass, K., Liebergott, J., & Swope, S. (1975). *Symbolic play in normal and language-impaired children.* Paper presented to the American Speech-Language-Hearing Association, Washington, DC.

Camarata, S., Newhoff, M., & Rugg, B. (1981, June). *Perspective taking in normal and language disordered children.* Paper presented at the Symposium of Research in Child Language Disorders, University of Wisconsin, Madison.

Camarata, S., Newhoff, M., & Rugg, B. (1985). Classification skills and language development in language impaired children. *Australian Journal of Human Communication Disorders, 13,* 107–115.

Ceci, S. (1983). Automatic and purposive semantic processing characteristics of normal and language/learning disabled children. *Developmental Psychology, 19,* 427–439.

Chi, M., & Gallagher, J. (1982). Speed of processing: A developmental source of limitation. *Topics in Learning and Learning Disabilities, 2,* 23–32.

Clahsen, H. (1989). The grammatical characterization of developmental aphasia. *Linguistics, 27,* 897–920.

Cromer, R. (1983). Hierarchical planning disability in the drawings and constructions of a special group of severely aphasic children. *Brain and Cognition, 2,* 144–164.

Doehring, D. (1960). Visual spatial memory in aphasic children. *Journal of Speech and Hearing Research, 3,* 138–149.

Eisenson, J. (1968). Developmental aphasia: A postulation of a unitary concept of the disorder. *Cortex, 4,* 184–200.

Ellis Weismer, S., Murray-Branch, J., & Miller, J. (1991, November). *Language development patterns in late talkers and typically developing children.* Paper presented at the annual convention of the American Speech-Language-Hearing Association, Atlanta, GA.

Farb, P. (1974). *Word play: What happens when people talk.* New York: Knopf.

Fazio, B. (1990). *Cognitive and linguistic factors associated with young language-impaired children's counting abilities.* Unpublished doctoral dissertation, Indiana University, Bloomington.

Inhelder, B. (1976). Observations on the operational and figurative aspects of thought in dysphasic children. In D. Morehead & A. Morehead (Eds.), *Normal and deficient child language.* Baltimore: University Park Press.

Johnston, J.R. (1988). Specific language disorders in the child. In N. Lass, L. McReynolds, J. Northerm, & D. Yoder (Eds.), *Handbook of speech-language pathology and audiology* (pp. 685–715). Toronto, Ontario, Canada: B.C. Decker.

Johnston, J.R., & Ellis Weismer, S. (1983). Mental rotation abilities in language-disordered children. *Journal of Speech and Hearing Research, 26,* 397–403.

Johnston, J.R., & Ramstad, V. (1983). Cognitive development in preadolescent language-impaired children. *British Journal of Disorders of Communication, 18,* 49–55.

Johnston, J.R., & Smith, L. (1988). *Six ways to skin a cat: Communication strategies used by language-impaired preschoolers.* Paper presented at the Symposium on Research in Child Language Disorders, University of Wisconsin, Madison.

Johnston, J.R., & Smith, L.B. (1989). Dimensional thinking in language impaired children. *Journal of Speech and Hearing Research, 32,* 33–38.

Kail, R., & Bisanz, J. (1982). Information processing and cognitive development. In L. Lipsitt & C. Spiker (Eds.), *Advances in child development and behavior* (Vol. 17). New York: Academic Press.

Kamhi, A., Gentry, B., & Mauer, D. (1990). Analogical learning and transfer in language-impaired children. *Journal of Speech and Hearing Disorders, 55,* 140–148.

Kamhi, A. (1981). Nonlinguistic symbolic and conceptual abilities of language-impaired and normally developing children. *Journal of Speech and Hearing Research, 24,* 446–453.

Kirchner, D., & Klatzky, R. (1985). Verbal rehearsal and memory in language-disordered children. *Journal of Speech and Hearing Research, 28,* 556–564.

Kosslyn, S. (1980). *Image and mind.* Cambridge, MA: Harvard University Press.

Kracke, I., (1975). Perception of rhythmic sequences by receptive aphasic and deaf children. *British Journal of Disorders of Communication, 10,* 43–51.

Leonard, L., Steckol, K., & Schwartz, R. (1978). Semantic relations and utterance length in child language. In F. Peng (Ed.), *Language acquisition and developmental kinesics* (pp. 93–107). Hiroshima: Bunka Hyoron.

Lovell, K., Hoyle, H., & Siddall, M. (1968). A study of some aspects of the play and language of young children with delayed speech. *Journal of Child Psychology & Psychiatry & Allied Disciplines, 3,* 41–50.

Lowe, M., & Costello, A. (1976). *The symbolic play test.* Windsor, England: NFER.-Nelson.

Mackworth, N., Grandstaff, N., & Pribram, K. (1973). Orientation to pictorial novelty by speech disordered children. *Neuropsychologia, 11,* 443–450.

Moore, M. (1990). *Adverbial and inflectional expressions of past time by normal and language-impaired children.* Unpublished doctoral dissertation, Indiana University, Bloomington.

Morehead, D. (1972). Early grammatical and semantic relations: Some implications for a general representational deficit in linguistically deviant children. *Papers and Reports on Child Language Development, 4,* 1–12.

Nelson, L.K., Kamhi, A.G., & Apel, K. (1987). Cognitive strengths and weaknesses in language-impaired children: One more look. *Journal of Speech and Hearing Disorders, 52,* 36–43.

Olson, D. (1975). On the relations between spatial and linguistic processes. In J. Eliot & N. Salkind (Eds.), *Children's spatial development* (pp. 67–110). Springfield, IL: Charles C Thomas.

Panagos, J., & Prelock, P. (1982). Phonological constraints on the sentence productions of language-disordered children. *Journal of Speech and Hearing Research, 25,* 536–547.

Pettito, L. (in press). The acquisition of sign in deaf children. In M. Gopnik (Ed.), *The biological basis of language,* London: Oxford University Press.

Pinker, S. (1989). Language acquisition. In M. Posner (Ed.), *Foundations of cognitive science.* Cambridge, MA: MIT Press.

Roth, F.P., & Clark, D.M. (1987). Symbolic play and social participation abilities of language-impaired and normally developing children. *Journal of Speech and Hearing Disorders, 52,* 17–29.

Saxe, G. (1979). Developmental relations between notational counting and number conversation. *Child Development, 50,* 180–187.

Schery, T. (1980). *Correlates of language development in language-disordered children: An archival study.* Unpublished doctoral dissertation, Claremont Graduate School, Claremont, CA.

Shore, C., Bates, E., Bretherton, I., Beeghly, M., & O'Connell, B. (1990). Vocal and gestural symbols: Similarities and differences from 13 to 28 months. In V. Volterra & C. Erting (Eds.), *From gesture to language in hearing and deaf children.* New York: Springer-Verlag.

Siegel, L., Lees, A., Allan, L., & Bolton, B. (1981). Nonverbal assessment of Piagetian concepts in preschool children with impaired language development. *Educational Psychology, 1,* 153–158.

Skarakis, E., & Prutting, C. (1988). Characteristics of symbolic play in language-disordered children. *Human Communication, 12,* 7–18.

Snyder, L. (1978). Communicative and cognitive abilities and disabilities in the sensorimotor period. *Merrill-Palmer Quarterly, 24,* 161–180.

Tallal, P. (1988). Research implication: A perspective. In R. Stark, P. Tallal, & R. McCauley (Eds.), *Language, speech and reading disorders in children* (pp. 160–168). Boston: Little, Brown.

Tallal, P. (1990). Fine-grained discrimination deficits in language-learning impaired children are specific neither to the auditory modality nor to speech perception. *Journal of Speech and Hearing Research, 33,* 616–617.

Tallal, P., & Piercy, M. (1973). Developmental aphasia: Impaired rate of nonverbal processing as a function of sensory modality. *Neuropsychologia, 11,* 389–398.

Tallal, P., Stark, R., Kallman, C., & Mellits, D. (1981). A reexamination of some nonverbal perceptual abilities of language impaired and normal children as a function of age and sensory modality. *Journal of Speech and Hearing Research, 24,* 351–357.

Terrell, B., & Schwartz, R. (1988). Object transformations in the play of language-impaired children. *Journal of Speech and Hearing Disorders, 53,* 459–466.

Terrell, B.Y., Schwartz, R.G., Prelock, P.A., & Messick, C.J. (1984). Symbolic play in normal and disordered children. *Journal of Speech and Hearing Research, 27,* 424–429.

Thal, D., & Bates, E. (1988). Language and gesture in late talkers. *Journal of Speech and Hearing Research, 31,* 115–123.

Udwin, O., & Yule, W. (1983). Imaginative play in language-disordered children. *British Journal of Disorders of Communication, 18,* 197–205.

Wyke, M., & Asso, D. (1979). Perception and memory for spatial relations in children with developmental dysphasia. *Neuropsychologia, 17,* 231–239.

8

Social Competence and Language Impairment in Children

Martin Fujiki and Bonnie Brinton

T RADITIONALLY, INTEREST IN CHILDREN WITH specific language impairment (SLI) has focused on the fact that these children do not reach linguistic milestones with the same ease as do their peers without impairments. More recently, the cognitive involvement and academic difficulties associated with language impairment have received considerable attention (e.g., see Johnston, chap. 7, and Catts, Hu, Larrivee, & Swank, chap. 9, this volume). However, the social functioning of children with SLI has typically been neglected in both research and clinical practice. This neglect is a matter of concern because it is widely recognized that children with a range of disabilities have difficulty with social interaction (Antia & Kreimeyer, 1992; Bryan, 1986; Guralnick, 1992). For example, Odom, McConnell, and Chandler (1990) (cited in Odom, McConnell, & McEvoy, 1992) reported that preschool teachers of special education classrooms indicated that 75% of their students needed to learn to participate more effectively in social interactions. Bryan observed that "the most consistent finding in learning disabilities research is that these children elicit negative judgments from others" (p. 229). Guralnick reported that, "Unfortunately, existing research has revealed that, overall, children with disabilities have a peer interaction deficit; that is, their degree of involvement in peer interactions falls substantially below expectations based on their developmental levels" (p. 56).

Considering the prevalence of social problems in children with a variety of disabilities, it might be expected that children with SLI would also be at risk for social difficulties. In fact, this risk is magnified because, by definition, children with SLI have limited communicative competence, and commu-

Preparation of this chapter was supported, in part, by a research grant from the College of Education, Brigham Young University.

nicative competence and social competence overlap to a significant degree (Prutting, 1982). Despite the high risk for social difficulties in children with SLI, researchers and clinicians have just begun to examine the social competence of these children (see Craig, 1993; Gallagher, 1991; Goldstein & Gallagher, 1992; Rice, 1993; in press; for discussion).

DEFINING SOCIAL COMPETENCE

Perhaps the place to begin a discussion of social competence is with a definition. However, this is not as simple as might be thought. Although social competence has been discussed by researchers representing a number of disciplines, there has been little agreement as to what social competence specifically involves (Dodge, 1985). As Siperstein (1992) noted, social competence has been defined to emphasize a variety of factors including appropriateness of interaction, amount of social interaction, demonstration of specific behaviors, and judgments of proficiency (both by self and others).

In the introduction to a recent issue of the *Journal of Applied Behavior Analysis* devoted to the topic of social competence, Odom and McConnell (1992) observed that the notions of effectiveness and appropriateness are prominent in many definitions of social competence (e.g., Guralnick, 1992; Odom et al., 1992). Thus, these authors proposed a definition based on earlier work by Foster and Ritchey (1979), stating that, "Social competence is the effective and appropriate use of social behavior in interactions with an individual or individuals" (p. 239). In this definition, the term *effective* implies that the behavior must result in a positive outcome for the individual. Thus, effective social behavior would improve interaction with others. Ineffective behavior would have the opposite result. To be "appropriate," the behavior must be suitable given the social context in which it is produced. For example, telling a joke may be acceptable in one social situation, but not another. As Odom and McConnell note, appropriateness is determined by a range of factors, including (but not limited to) "the specific social circumstances, and the social norms or values of the participants" (p. 240).

Although the definition proposed by Odom and McConnell (1992) has certain limitations, it provides a useful point of reference in discussing children with SLI. In the following sections, we first discuss the importance of social competence to the study of children with SLI. We then review some findings regarding the social competence of these children. Finally, we suggest several clinical implications based on these data.

IMPORTANCE OF SOCIAL COMPETENCE TO CHILDREN WITH SLI

Examining social competence is important to the study of children with SLI for at least two reasons: 1) the development of social competence and communicative competence are closely related, and 2) there is a high correlation between language impairment and problematic socioemotional behavior.

Development of Social Competence and Communicative Competence

The relationship between certain aspects of social behavior and language behavior has been the subject of a fair amount of investigation. For example, the influence of caregiver–infant interaction on language development has been examined by numerous authors (e.g., Snow, 1984; Snow & Ferguson, 1977). However, less attention has been focused on the association between language acquisition, social skills, and socioemotional development. Although the specific role that social interaction plays in the language acquisition process (and vice versa) is a subject of debate, it is clear that the development of social interaction and the acquisition of language are not independent phenomena.

Prizant and Wetherby (1990) observed that there appear to be both "mutual influences and interdependencies" between aspects of social development and language development. This point was illustrated by Berko Gleason, Hay, and Cain (1989) in their discussion of the literature on early language development. These authors noted that in the first weeks of life, infants make affective and social distinctions, showing an interest in human faces and preferring their mothers' voices. Caregivers respond by treating early infant vocalizations as if they had communicative intent, in essence, building conversations around infants' contributions. These early exchanges provide a fertile context for the acquisition of language, and, at the same time, contribute to the development and maintenance of attachments between infants and caregivers. As children develop, a need for social interaction characterizes such early communicative acts as directing the behavior of others (e.g., requesting) and maintaining social contact (e.g., showing objects). Berko Gleason et al. contended that it is an inherent human need for social interaction that stimulates early linguistic production. At the same time, a basic function of language is to "sustain and maintain emotional attachments that are common to human beings at every stage in their lives" (Berko Gleason et al., 1989, p. 172). As children develop from infancy to the preschool years and then beyond, the interrelationship of language and social domains continues to be strong (see Prizant & Wetherby, 1990, for additional discussion).

Although a relationship between language and social domains is evident, the nature of this association has been difficult to describe. It is tempting to think of linguistic and social behaviors in terms of direct causality. For example, a poor social environment might result in poor language skills, or conversely, poor language skills might preclude the development of appropriate social skills. However, the relationship between social competence and communicative competence is probably too complex to be viewed in this manner.

Sameroff and Chandler (1975) described a transactional model of development that provides a helpful framework to consider how linguistic and social aspects of human relationships are intertwined. This transactional model is particularly useful in contemplating the interrelationship of language impairment, problematic social skills, and more serious socioemotional difficulties.

In the transactional model, development is viewed as resulting from the "continuous dynamic interactions of the child and the experience provided by his or her family and social context" (Sameroff, 1987, p. 278). Thus, behavior at any particular point in time is not viewed as the result of a specific event or influence, but rather as the result of the ongoing interactions between child, caregiver, and environment. Emphasis is placed on the mutual potency of the child and the social environment to influence each other in a dynamic manner.

Viewed from a transactional perspective, a child's social and language functioning are influenced by characteristics inherent to the child as well as by his or her cumulative social experiences. Children bring certain attributes to the task of language acquisition. For example, from infancy, humans process auditory stimuli in a way that suggests a propensity to attend to important linguistic features. At the same time, the social environment provides the context that will cultivate or discourage the development of these propensities. Thus, social experiences affect the development of language, and language skills influence the social environment in an ongoing, dynamic way. For example, Sameroff (Sameroff, 1987; Sameroff & Fiese, 1990) presented an illustration of how parental anxiety regarding a complicated birth might result in a series of events in the behavior of both mother and infant, ultimately leading to reduced interaction and negative influences on language development. Consider a similar illustration emphasizing the interrelationship of the social environment and language impairment. A toddler with SLI has particular difficulty responding to maternal linguistic input. Because the child frequently appears to be nonresponsive, the mother finds that interacting with the child is not enjoyable, and unconsciously reduces the amount of time spent interacting with the child. This reduced interaction results in fewer opportunities for the child to participate in social exchanges. Assuming that experience is important in developing social and linguistic skills, decreased social exchanges negatively influence both the child's social and linguistic development.

In our own work, we have observed numerous examples that emphasize the interrelationship of social and communicative competence. Consider the case of a 4-year-old boy with documented language impairment referred to as P. P's language comprehension was mildly to moderately depressed, and his production was markedly impaired. His speech was characterized by numerous phonological errors, which reduced intelligibility dramatically. His productive syntax was limited to short, simple utterances, and his morphological system was immature. In addition, P typically did not interact with children outside his family. We observed P in a neighborhood play context for several months. Initially, neighborhood peers attempted to include P in their play. However, P had difficulty initiating appropriate exchanges with other children and responding appropriately to their bids to interact. In one instance, shortly after P and a neighborhood peer had met, the peer approached P to engage him in play. P yelled, "Go away!" The peer attempted to negotiate ("You still want me to go away?") and approached P several times. P continued to yell "Go away!" In other instances, P played independently while other children played around him. P did not take part in group play scripts such as "playing house." Only once did we note a felicitous, interactive exchange with children other than his sisters. (This exchange involved P, a 2-year-old girl, and a 4-year-old boy. These children played a game in which they alternately hit each other on the head with a diaper and then laughed hysterically.) Although P seemed to like children in the neighborhood (he sometimes spontaneously hugged a peer), he continued to reject most of their social bids. On one occasion, we asked P and the 4-year-old peer mentioned previously to interact in our laboratory setting. Throughout the interaction, neither P nor the peer was consistently responsive to the other. At one point, P presented a compelling bid, "I got new doggie. Want come my house see it?" The peer ignored the bid, perhaps because he found it unintelligible, or perhaps because he had grown unresponsive to P. P did not attempt to repair or reissue the bid, and an opportunity for a meaningful exchange was lost.

This instance provided a glimpse into the relationship between P's limited communicative competence and his social ineptitude. P's case is illustrative of what Rice (in press) has described as the social consequences account of language impairment. P's language skills limited his ability to engage his peers in conversation, and his social skills restricted his language environment. P tended to reject the social and conversational bids of his peers, and his peers grew to ignore him in group or dyadic play. P's social needs were not well served by his communicative skills, and his opportunities to use language for communication were constrained by his social skills. Clearly, P's social and communicative functioning were intertwined in very real ways.

In summary, the linguistic environment of a young child is distinctly social, and language usage may have an important influence on the manner in which the child is perceived and related to by caregivers and peers. In addition, the child's social environment is likely to influence the development of linguistic skills. Viewed from a transactional perspective, a child's language and social functioning are mutually influential in a dynamic manner.

Relationship Between Problematic Socioemotional Behavior and Language Impairment

The relationship between language impairment, social problems, and more serious socioemotional difficulties is complex. It is possible to hypothesize a number of associations. For example, language impairment might hinder the development of appropriate social skills, which would lead to difficulty in the development of social relationships. These problems might eventually lead to the development of more serious socioemotional impairment. However, it is likely that the relationship between these problems is more complex than this example suggests, with a disorder in one area interacting with and intensifying problems in other areas. In this section, we focus on the relationship between language impairment and various types of problematic socioemotional behaviors.

The relationship between aspects of language behavior and certain types of socially challenging behaviors is well accepted in the study of developmental disabilities. For instance, it has been demonstrated that for many persons with mental retardation, such challenging behaviors as noncompliance, self-injury, and physical aggression are avenues to express communicative intent (e.g., the desire to gain attention or to avoid an aversive task) (Carr & Durand, 1985; Donnellan, Mirenda, Mesaros, & Fassbender, 1984). This notion has stimulated the development of innovative intervention programs that provide the individual with more acceptable alternatives for communicating these intentions (e.g., Carr, 1982; Reichle & Johnston, 1993).

The relationship between problematic social behavior and communicative competence appears to be significant in higher functioning populations as well. A number of studies have reported a high incidence of language impairment in populations defined by the presence of problematic socioemotional behavior. For example, Camarata, Hughes, and Ruhl (1988) found a high incidence of language impairment in children with mild-to-moderate behavior disorders. Thirty-seven of thirty-eight subjects showed some evidence of language impairment as measured by formal testing. Miniutti (1991) reported that inner-city children with behavior problems had significantly lower language scores on the Clinical Evaluation of Language Fundamentals–Revised (Semel, Wiig, & Secord, 1987) than a chronological age–matched group of control subjects. Baltaxe and Simmons (1991) found a high incidence of communication problems in conjunction with a wide range of psychiatric disorders, across a range of age groups. Numerous other reports have also discussed relationships between speech and/or language impairment and socioemotional behavior (e.g., Baker & Cantwell, 1982; 1987a, 1987b; Baltaxe & Simmons, 1988a, 1988b; Beitchman, 1985; Cantwell & Baker, 1987; Davis, Sanger, & Morris-Friehe, 1991; Mack & Warr-Leeper, 1992; Prizant & Wetherby, 1990; Prizant et al., 1990).

One line of research that is illustrative of this relationship was reported by Baker and Cantwell (1982; 1987a, 1987b). These researchers performed psychiatric evaluations on 600 children seen at a community speech and hearing clinic for a speech evaluation. Of these children, approximately 50% (302) received psychiatric diagnoses. Baker and Cantwell (1987b) retested

300 (of the original 600) subjects approximately 5 years after their initial assessments. The follow-up psychiatric evaluations revealed an increase in psychiatric diagnoses, from 44% (of the 300 subjects retested) to 60%. Baker and Cantwell noted that most of the children developing psychiatric problems showed some type of behavior problem, including attention deficits and anxiety disorders.

In considering several possible explanations of these findings, Baker and Cantwell (1987a) suggest that it is likely that communication problems contribute to the development of psychiatric impairment. Baker and Cantwell state that "communication difficulties produce a variety of psychosocial deficits, which in turn may be mechanisms for the development of psychiatric disorders" (p. 195). They also point out that there are several other ways in which communication problems might lead to psychiatric difficulties. For example, it might be hypothesized that communication problems would lead to difficulty in establishing the peer relationships important to normal childhood social development.

Regardless of whether one type of impairment leads to another, such data as those presented by Baker and Cantwell (1987a, 1987b) emphasize the high cooccurrence of these problems. There is little doubt that many socioemotional problems are displayed in language use, and that performance on a number of language parameters contributes to the identification and labeling of behaviors considered to be deviant.

SOCIAL COMPETENCE OF CHILDREN WITH SLI

Successful social interactions and successful social relationships in childhood are influenced by a range of skills, many of which are linguistically manifest (e.g., Black & Hazen, 1990; Gottman, 1983; Hazen & Black, 1989; Place & Becker, 1991). Because of the critical role of language in most social interactions, it is likely that children with SLI are at risk for social failure. However, the literature on the social competence of these children is incomplete. There has been a good deal of study focusing on the pragmatic skills of these children, as well as on the interactions between children with SLI and their caregivers. Nevertheless, our knowledge of the wider social ramifications of language impairment is limited. For example, a number of studies have suggested that some children with SLI have difficulty with specific aspects of conversational management (e.g., Brinton & Fujiki, 1982; Conti-Ramsden & Friel-Patti, 1983; Craig & Evans, 1989). Although these studies have provided insights into the manner in which children with SLI interact, there are few empirical data documenting how deficits in conversational skill influence the social relationships of these children (e.g., the ability to make and keep friends). The following is a review of several studies that have direct and indirect implications for the social relationships of children with SLI. In discussing these studies, we have focused on three overlapping aspects of social behavior. First, we discuss briefly the social tasks that children with SLI must perform. We then review several studies documenting socially penalizing linguistic behaviors that these children have produced. Finally, we examine the social reactions they receive from their peers.

Social Tasks Confronting Children with SLI

A number of researchers have emphasized the importance of the social task or situation in assessing social competence (e.g., Dodge, Pettit, McClaskey, & Brown, 1986). There has been a good deal of research studying the ability of typically developing children to perform specific types of social tasks, such as initiating interaction, accessing an ongoing exchange, and managing a confrontation. Given the cognitive and sensory status of children with SLI, it is probable that the social tasks that they must perform are similar to those performed by their peers without impairments. However, information on the ability of children with SLI to perform various types of social tasks is relatively limited.

In one of the few studies of its kind involving children with SLI, Craig and Washington (1993) examined the ability of five subjects with SLI and their language and chronological age–matched peers to access, or enter, an ongoing dyadic interaction. It was observed that all the children in both control groups were able to enter the ongoing play quickly. However, three of the children with SLI were unable to access the interaction during a 20-minute observation period. The remaining two children did so only with nonverbal behaviors.

In a discussion of an individual subject with SLI performing the same task, Craig (1993) observed that the child, Gary, appeared hesitant to join the ongoing interaction upon entering the room. Gary did not approach the children, but stopped and observed the interaction from a distance, saying, "I'll stand here." It was of interest that Gary did not even employ one of the more basic strategies used by children without SLI to gain access, that of placing himself in close proximity to the ongoing interaction (e.g., Corsaro, 1985).

In another study, Gallagher and Craig (1984) presented research that described a child who used an unusual tactic to initiate and access interaction. These authors described a 4-year-old boy with SLI, Clark, who frequently used the phrase "It's gone (IG)." Detailed analysis of interactions revealed that Clark's use of "IG" was semantically appropriate to context and functioned as a bid to engage his conversational partner in a "nonexistence/ disappearance" game. Gallagher and Craig point out that in the interaction of mothers and very young children without disabilities, this type of game commonly provides a positive interactional context with relatively few linguistic demands on the child. Clark played this game with his mother, which resulted in a positive social interaction for both participants. However, attempts to engage other partners in the game, using the phrase "IG" as a means of inviting interaction, were much less successful. On most occasions, the phrase did not result in initiation of the game or in maintaining interaction. Most often, the other child ignored Clark.

These reports provide strong preliminary evidence that children with SLI may have difficulty performing some of the basic social tasks they face. Further research examining the ability of these children to negotiate these basic social tasks is needed.

Socially Penalizing Linguistic Behaviors in Children with SLI

As noted previously, there are numerous studies documenting the coexistence of problematic social behaviors and language impairment in persons with a range of disabilities. Regarding children with SLI, there are also reports documenting pragmatic deficits that would have the potential to produce negative social consequences. Additionally, recent work has demonstrated that the presence of speech and language impairment negatively influences adults' perception of children across several domains (Burroughs & Tomblin, 1990; Rice, Hadley, & Alexander, in press). All this work could be included in a discussion of socially penalizing behaviors. However, we have narrowed our focus to specific instances in which linguistic behaviors directly resulted in social problems for children. As such, all the studies reviewed focus on individual subjects and negative social reactions that are documented by reports of persons interacting with those individuals. We have also limited our discussion to children who, from the available information, are described by the term *SLI,* rather than by autism or mental retardation.

Tomblin and Liljegreen (1985) reported the case of Marcia, a 12-year-old female with a range of language problems. Marcia had received speech-language pathology services since the age of 4. At the time she was seen by Tomblin and Liljegreen, she was enrolled in a residential treatment facility for children with communication disabilities. Staff members were asked to keep logs noting instances in which Marcia's communication problems resulted in social problems with others. Based on these observations, two communication problems were identified as being most problematic: a low rate of responsiveness and a high frequency of complaining. It was notable, but not surprising, that of the range of linguistic deficits demonstrated, the two behaviors identified by staff were social in nature. In further assessment of her responsiveness, it was found that Marcia frequently did not respond to the requests or comments of others, and when she did reply, the response was often minimal. Further study revealed that Marcia's nonresponsiveness appeared to be linked to topic manipulation. She appeared capable of interacting on topics that she had initiated, but was nonresponsive to topics initiated by others.

Fujiki and Brinton (1991) described a child with SLI who was characterized by the rather unusual pattern of being highly assertive and moderately responsive in conversation. This child, referred to as H, was a highly outgoing, verbal child. Because of this, his teachers frequently overestimated his ability to handle linguistic material. However, they were fully aware of his general academic problems. Furthermore, his classroom teacher and other school personnel reported that he was a *different* child, who had difficulty in social interactions with peers. H was observed in interactions with a language age–matched (LA) peer, a chronological age–matched (CA) peer, and an adult. In each of these interactions, H talked more than his conversational partner, producing 62%, 77%, and 71% of the utterances in the interaction with the adult, CA peer, and LA peer, respectively. In each of these interactions, he was responsible for approximately 75% of the total number of assertions produced by both speakers. In the peer interactions, he was responsible for over 80% of the requests produced. H introduced a large number of topics; however, many of these topics were not maintained by the dyad. On occasion, the topic introduced by H seemed irrelevant to the current context. Although H produced a large number of requests, it was notable that most of these were not requests for information, but bids to retain the speaking floor.

It is difficult to quantify the degree to which H's interactional style contributed to his problems interacting with peers. However, it is suspected that his conversational pattern was related to his difficulties in establishing relationships and making friends. Both of H's peer partners made comments during the course of the interaction that indicated their awareness of and annoyance with his conversational style.

In the Gallagher and Craig (1984) study discussed previously, Clark's frequent use of "It's gone" could also be considered as a socially penalizing behavior. As noted previously, the overuse of this phrase served to confuse and frustrate the children with whom Clark interacted. Goldstein and Gallagher (1992) reported that following the conclusion of the Gallagher and Craig study, Clark was enrolled in an intervention program. One of the goals of intervention was to replace "It's gone" with a socially more appropriate phrase that would serve a similar function. The phrase, "Let's play," was selected. Goldstein and Gallagher noted that this produced a positive response from peers and resulted in decreased use of "It's gone."

Brinton and Fujiki (in press) presented a detailed study of a 6-year-old child with SLI. CD exhibited a number of linguistic strengths and weaknesses. He had notable difficulty with complex syntactic forms and vocabulary items. However, his phonological skills were relatively good, and he was appropriately assertive in conversation. However, in certain situations he was not as responsive as was desirable. Clinical goals included responding appropriately to the questions of others, discussing topics outside of current context, producing complex sentences, and increasing the range of vocabulary items.

Of interest in the current discussion was CD's use of the term *liar*. For example, when CD asked for milk, his mother told him that there was some in the refrigerator. When CD looked in the refrigerator he could not see any milk, and responded, "Liar." CD began using this term with a number of individuals both at home and at school, almost always eliciting negative responses. After analysis of the contexts in which this word was used, it was determined that CD was using this term to mean, "You made a mistake." In order to deal with this behavior, CD's mother and clinician agreed to handle occurrences of "liar" in a similar manner. When CD used this term, the person he was speaking to would state, "I feel bad when you say liar to me." An alternative form was then modeled. With implementation of this strategy, the inappropriate use of the term *liar* soon disappeared.

Reports such as these indicate that children with SLI sometimes use their language skills in ways that may elicit social penalties from others. Furthermore, these difficulties extend beyond the types of penalties that might initially come to mind (e.g., teasing from peers, negative comments about unintelligible speech).

Peer Reactions to Children with SLI

Peer reactions are closely related to penalizing behaviors that children with SLI demonstrate. A number of researchers have reported impressions by the teachers and peers of children with SLI that indicate, at least in those individual instances, negative social reactions (Brinton & Fujiki, 1989; Craig, 1993; McTear, 1985; Rice, 1993). For example, Craig reports the comment of a typically developing child shortly after meeting a child with SLI; "That kid's strange!"

There are also empirical data suggesting that children are aware of the speech and language abilities of their peers with SLI, and respond differently to them. For example, Craig and Gallagher (1986) examined the frequency with which typically developing conversational partners of differing ages responded to the comments of a 4-year-old with SLI (Clark). It was found that 2;6-year-old partners responded to Clark's comments with related responses at about the same rate that they responded to the comments of both other 2;6- and 4-year-old typically developing partners. However, the 4-year-olds responded to Clark's comments at about one half the rate that they responded to the comments of 2;6-year-olds and 4-year-olds.

A number of revealing studies have been conducted by Rice and her colleagues, working in the Language Acquisition Preschool at the University of Kansas. These researchers have reported several projects examining the interactional skills of children with language impairment. For example, Rice,

Sell, and Hadley (1991) examined the interactions of four groups of children in a preschool setting. These groups included children 1) who were developing typically, 2) with language impairments (LI), 3) with speech impairments (SI), and 4) who were learning English as a second language (ESL). Conversational turns produced during play time were coded as to function (initiations or responses) and addressee. It was found that typically developing children preferred other typically developing children as partners. Furthermore, children with normal skills were the preferred addressee for all groups of children. Children with SI and LI preferred to initiate interaction with adults. The ESL children were the least likely to initiate interaction, and were the least preferred addressees of the other children. These findings suggest that the children were aware of their own communication abilities, as well as the communication skills of others, at a relatively young age. Moreover, this knowledge appeared to influence their selection of conversational partners.

Rice et al. (1991) speculated that patterns of interaction between children might be influenced by conversational responsiveness. For example, it might be expected that children would direct a majority of their initiations to those conversational partners who were most responsive. In order to investigate this possibility, Hadley and Rice (1991) examined the responsiveness of various groups of children in the language acquisition preschool setting. In this investigation, subjects were separated into groups of LI, SI, marginal impairment, and typical language.

The groups did not significantly differ in the total number of interactions or conversational turns in which they participated. However, children with marginal and normal language abilities spent a higher proportion of their time interacting with peers than did children with impairments. In peer interactions, it was found that the initiations of children in the SI and LI groups were frequently ignored by peers, and that these children responded less often when a peer initiated an interaction with them. Because responsiveness is a basic requirement for successful conversational interaction, it is likely that this lack of responsiveness would be a significant hindrance. Based on these and other similar data, Rice (1993; in press) has suggested that young children with SLI may be in danger of "a negative social spiral." Rice suggested that children with speech and or language disabilities initially may lack the linguistic skills needed to participate actively in social interactions with their peers. Therefore, they may be less liked by their peers and experience a high rate of rejection. They may also develop compensatory behaviors, such as directing most of their initiations to adults or shortening their utterances.

In addition to the issues discussed above, there is another aspect of peer reaction that merits discussion. It has been recognized for some time that the conversational behaviors used by speakers are mutually influential (e.g., Feldstein & Welkowitz, 1978). The poor interactional skills demonstrated by children with SLI may have a particularly negative influence on the conversational behavior of their partners. Consider the child described in the Fujiki and Brinton (1991) study, referred to as H. As was noted, H was observed in interactions with a LA peer, a CA peer, and an adult. In both peer interactions, it was of interest to note that both the LA and the CA peer became less responsive as the interaction progressed. Thus, on the surface, it would appear that H's peers were relatively nonresponsive, responding to approximately 50% of his requests. Even the adult responded to only 75% of H's requests. However, H's peers and the adult did not demonstrate this pattern in other interactions. Rather, this nonresponsive style of interaction appeared to be a response to H's interactional style. It might be speculated that as H's conversational partners became more annoyed or frustrated by his attempts to dominate the conversation, they also became less interactive.

Further research is needed to clarify our understanding of the social competence of children with SLI. Preliminary research on the social consequences of language impairment suggests that children with SLI often do elicit negative reactions from their peers and participate in fewer positive interactions with peers.

CLINICAL IMPLICATIONS

Consideration of the relationship between communicative competence and social competence lends credence to the conclusion that SLI is not an isolated deficit as was once envisioned. Rather, language functioning seems to be closely tied with social functioning in complex and dynamic ways. Research on structural and pragmatic language deficits must be expanded to consider the impact of these impairments on the individual's social world. At the same time, clinical approaches to language impairment must be stretched to deal with social aspects of interaction and with the influence of social factors on language. Furthermore, efforts to teach social skills independent of language abilities, or vice versa, are ill advised.

We have formulated a few points that we feel are important in the assessment and intervention of children with SLI in light of the previous discussion.

1. *Language impairment and social deficits may be inextricably intertwined in a variety of different ways.* As we have stressed throughout this chapter, language impairment may heighten social difficulties, and social problems may perpetuate language impairment. As Gallagher (1991) noted, "speech-language pathologists need to become more concerned about the social aspects of language disorders because they may be inherent to language disorder and/or may contribute as precipitating and maintaining factors" (p. 34). In addition to addressing problems of language form, content, and use, the treatment of language impairment must also include provision for social elements that may be inherent to or associated with communicative disorders.

On a related note, it is important to remember that in some children with SLI, these social problems may be related to more serious socioemotional difficulties. In working with these children, the speech-language pathologist may play a key role in obtaining and providing appropriate clinical services. In many cases, the speech-language pathologist will be the first or the only professional to see a child with these difficulties. In making referrals, it is critical to work with other professionals to develop an appropriate treatment plan. Careful coordination of services is necessary to address the child's needs effectively. As noted by Prizant et al. (1990), it is also important for the speech-language pathologist to educate parents and professionals about the nature of the communication impairment and the importance of approaching children with linguistic and socioemotional problems in a holistic manner. Without such efforts, intervention is likely to be fragmented and ultimately ineffective. The reader is referred to Prizant et al. (1990) and Hummel and Prizant (1993) for further discussion and elaboration on these issues.

2. *The ultimate success of intervention is determined by the child's ability to communicate with those persons in his or her social environment.* Traditionally, clinicians have focused their attention on how the client communicates within the clinical setting. Facilitating techniques are applied primarily in the context of the child's interaction with the clinician. Yet, the child's relatively cursory association with the clinician does not typically form a major social relationship. The true success of clinical intervention is determined by how the client communicates with the people most central to his or her social world (Johnston, 1985; Lyon, 1992; Rice, 1986).

Tomblin and Liljegreen (1985) stress the importance of implementing *socially relevant goals* in intervention. We contend that socially relevant goals are important to facilitate participation in conversations in a way that helps to establish and maintain relationships with adults and peers. This philosophy will stretch the context of language intervention to include not only the child with language impairment, but also a wide variety of conversational partners. In this regard, work with the child's family and other persons in the child's social environment is critical. As Sameroff and Fiese (1990) have observed in reference to early childhood intervention, efforts directed toward the child alone are almost certain to fail. We believe this is true in the case of children with SLI as well. It will be critical to involve the people in the child's family and social environments if intervention is to be most effective.

The notion of involving parents and others in the child's environment in intervention is not new, and a fair amount of information is readily available on this topic (e.g., MacDonald, 1989). However, one point that merits mention was suggested by Rice (1993). Rice presented data indicating that children with impaired speech and language skills are likely to be judged negatively on a range of abilities (e.g., cognitive ability, academic potential).

These negative judgments may have far-reaching academic and social consequences. Thus, Rice suggested that it may be possible to work with family
members as well as with other professionals working with the child to counter
misconceptions and mistaken impressions. Information regarding the nature
of language impairment in general, as well as the child's individual strengths
and weaknesses, may help to provide a better understanding of the child's
impairment.

   3. *Social intervention should be conducted early in development.*   In
the earlier discussion of the transactional model of development, it was emphasized that behavior at any particular point in time is the result of ongoing
interactions between child, caregiver, and environment. Therefore, early intervention can most effectively facilitate both linguistic and social development before negative patterns become long established. As Prizant and
Wetherby (1990) have suggested, early language intervention with children
and their families may help to avoid "the development or exacerbation of
emotional and behavioral problems" (p. 3).

   Early intervention is not only of importance with regard to parents and
other adults. Odom et al. (1992) note it is important to provide the child with
support in peer interactions before negative interactions establish the child's
reputation. This importance is underscored by data suggesting that the social
structure of the peer group becomes more rigid as the child enters the middle
childhood years (e.g., Howes,1990), which may make social interventions
more difficult.

   4. *It is important to consider the social ramifications of the linguistic
behaviors that we facilitate in intervention.*   This issue has several facets.
First, it is important to target behaviors in intervention that will empower the
child in social contexts. Intervention objectives should be designed to help the
child achieve his or her ends in conversation in socially acceptable ways.
Second, it is important to provide a supportive social environment in which to
use newly trained skills. Goldstein and Gallagher (1992) have suggested that
strategies that encourage the child to use new skills as well as strategies that
reinforce skills after they are used are desirable. Third, it is important to
consider the effects of targeted behaviors on others in the child's environment.
Adults and children who habitually converse with a child may be accustomed
to that child's interactional style. For example, if a child has traditionally been
reticent in conversation, more assertive behaviors trained in intervention may
startle his or her long-time conversational partners. It is our experience that it
is sometimes necessary to help the child's interactants accept and value new,
more independent, behaviors.

   5. *Conversational responsiveness in interactions is critical to social
relationships.*   A number of the research studies discussed have suggested
that an individual's responsiveness in conversation is critical to how that
person is perceived by conversational partners. In our own work, we have

found that responsiveness seems to have a direct impact on a speaker's social acceptance (e.g., Brinton & Fujiki, 1993). Specifically, conversational partners tend to prefer interacting with individuals responsive to their conversational contributions. Behaviors that convey interest in the feelings and needs of others foster the formation and maintenance of relationships.

Conversely, behaviors such as ignoring partners' conversational bids, failing to maintain topics introduced by others, and disregarding questions from others elicit negative social reactions. We have observed that a speaker who is not responsive to partners seems to elicit nonresponsive behaviors from those partners, resulting in mutually nonresponsive dyads (Fujiki & Brinton, 1991).

We would contend that facilitating conversational responsiveness is an important focus in intervention with those children who demonstrate nonresponsive behaviors. Facilitating conversational responsiveness has the potential to make the child more attractive as a conversational partner, to improve the child's language environment, and to enhance the child's social relationships.

6. *It is important to identify and replace socially penalizing behaviors.* As discussed previously, children with SLI may produce linguistic behaviors that elicit penalties from others. Goldstein and Gallagher (1992) have suggested that these behaviors should be identified and replaced by behaviors that serve similar functions but do not elicit similar negative reactions from others. The substitution of the phrase "Let's play" for "It's gone" in the language production of the child referred to as Clark (reported earlier) is an example of this procedure. Although these phrases were functionally equivalent, the use of the unconventional form "It's gone" as a bid to play often caused confusion or annoyance, and frequently did not produce the result Clark desired. "Let's play" was more acceptable to Clark's peers and was much more successful in achieving Clark's desired goal.

Goldstein and Gallagher (1992) suggest that these behaviors may be identified by observation. The negative impressions of those individuals who typically interact with the child may also be helpful in focusing the assessment. Care should be taken to determine if specific communicative behaviors are influential in creating negative impressions of the child. If this is the case, efforts should be made to provide the child with a more acceptable means of communicating. For example, if it is determined that a child uses physically aggressive acts to communicate his or her intent to escape from a work situation, a more acceptable means of communicating this intent might be substituted.

It should be considered that, as Goldstein and Gallagher (1992) point out, if the penalizing behavior does serve a communicative function, it will be ineffective, if not impossible, to simply eliminate it. Even if the form could be eliminated (e.g., making the child stop saying "It's gone"), the communicative need that the form served would remain.

SUMMARY

Social competence of children with SLI is an important area of study. Social competence and communicative competence overlap to the extent that neither can be well understood if the other is not considered. We are just beginning to appreciate the far-reaching effects of language impairment on a child's social functioning. At the same time, we are just beginning to explore the impact of socioemotional factors on a child's communicative skill. However, current research has already indicated that the relationship between social problems and language impairment is complex and cannot be described as a simple matter of causality.

The association between social competence and communicative competence in children has important ramifications for language intervention. Further research and clinical work are necessary to describe fully what those ramifications are. For now, we can assume that language impairment is not an isolated phenomenon, and should not be addressed as one clinically. Rather, the interplay between communicative, social, and other behaviors should form the focus for remediation.

REFERENCES

Antia, S.D., & Kreimeyer, K.H. (1992). Social competence intervention for young children with hearing impairments. In S.L. Odom, S.R. McConnell, & M.A. McEvoy (Eds.), *Social competence of young children with disabilities: Issues and strategies for intervention* (pp. 135–164). Baltimore: Paul H. Brookes Publishing Co.

Baker, L., & Cantwell, D.P. (1982). Language acquisition, cognitive development, and emotional disorder in childhood. In K.E. Nelson (Ed.), *Children's language* (Vol. 3, pp. 286–321). Hillsdale, NJ: Lawrence Erlbaum Associates.

Baker, L., & Cantwell, D.P. (1987a). Comparison of well, emotionally disordered, and behaviorally disordered children with linguistic problems. *Journal/of/the American Academy of Child and Adolescent Psychiatry, 26,* 193–196.

Baker, L., & Cantwell, D.P. (1987b). A prospective psychiatric follow-up of children with speech/language disorders. *Journal of the American Academy of Child and Adolescent Psychiatry, 26,* 546–553.

Baltaxe, C.A.M., & Simmons, J.Q. (1988a). Communication deficits in preschool children with psychiatric disorders. *Seminars in Speech and Language, 9,* 81–91.

Baltaxe, C.A.M., & Simmons, J.Q. (1988b). Pragmatic deficits in emotionally disturbed children and adolescents. In R.L. Schiefelbusch & L.L. Lloyd (Eds.), *Language perspectives: Acquisition, retardation, and intervention* (2nd ed., pp. 223–253). Austin, TX: PRO-ED.

Baltaxe, C.A.M., & Simmons, J.Q. (1991, November). *Communication disorders in five age groups of children and adolescents with psychiatric disorders.* Paper presented at the annual convention of the American Speech-Language-Hearing Association, Atlanta, GA.

Beitchman, J.H. (1985). Speech and language impairment and psychiatric risk: Toward a model of neurodevelopmental immaturity. *Psychiatric Clinics of North America, 8,* 721–735.

Berko Gleason, J., Hay, D., & Cain, L. (1989). Social and affective determinants of language acquisition. In M.L. Rice & R.L. Schiefelbusch (Eds.), *The teachability of language* (pp. 171–186). Baltimore: Paul H. Brookes Publishing Co.

Black, B., & Hazen, N.L. (1990). Social status and patterns of communication in acquainted and unacquainted preschool children. *Developmental Psychology, 26,* 379–387.

Brinton, B., & Fujiki, M. (1982). A comparison of request–response sequences in the discourse of normal and language-disordered children. *Journal of Speech and Hearing Disorders, 47,* 57–62.

Brinton, B., & Fujiki, M. (1989). *Conversational management with language-impaired children.* Rockville, MD: Aspen Publishers Inc.

Brinton, B., & Fujiki, M. (1993). Communication skills and community integration in adults with mild-to-moderate retardation. *Topics in Language Disorders, 13*(3), 9–19.

Brinton, B., & Fujiki, M. (in press). Conversational intervention with children with language impairment. In M.E. Fey, J. Windsor, & S.F. Warren (Eds.), *Communication and language intervention series: Vol. 5. Language intervention: Preschool through the primary school years.* Baltimore: Paul H. Brookes Publishing Co.

Bryan, T. (1986). A review of studies on learning-disabled children's communicative competence. In R.L. Schiefelbusch (Ed.), *Language competence: Assessment and intervention* (pp. 227–259). San Diego: College-Hill Press.

Burroughs, E.I., & Tomblin, J.B. (1990). Speech and language correlates of adults' judgments of children. *Journal of Speech and Hearing Disorders, 55,* 485–494.

Camarata, S.M., Hughes, C.A., & Ruhl, K.L. (1988). Mild/moderate behaviorally disordered students: A population at risk for language disorders. *Language, Speech and Hearing Services in Schools, 19,* 191–200.

Cantwell, D.P., & Baker, L. (1987). *Developmental speech and language disorders.* New York: Guilford Press.

Carr, E.G. (1982). *How to teach sign language to developmentally disabled children.* Lawrence, KS: H & H Enterprises.

Carr, E.G., & Durand, V.M. (1985). The social-communicative basis of severe behavior problems in children. In S. Reiss & R.R. Bootzin (Eds.), *Theoretical issues in behavior therapy* (pp. 219–254). New York: Academic Press.

Conti-Ramsden, G., & Friel-Patti, S. (1983). Mothers' discourse adjustments to language-impaired and nonlanguage-impaired children. *Journal of Speech and Hearing Disorders, 48,* 360–367.

Corsaro, W.A. (1985). *Friendship and peer culture in the early years.* Norwood, NJ: Ablex Publishing Co.

Craig, H.K. (1993). Social skills of children with specific language impairment: Peer relationships. *Language, Speech and Hearing Services in Schools, 24,* 206–215.

Craig, H.K., & Evans, J. (1989). Turn exchange characteristics of SLI childrens' simultaneous and nonsimultaneous speech. *Journal of Speech and Hearing Disorders, 54,* 334–347.

Craig, H.K., & Gallagher, T.M. (1986). Interactive play: The frequency of related verbal responses. *Journal of Speech and Hearing Research, 29,* 375–383.

Craig, H.K., & Washington, J.A. (1993). The access behaviors of children with specific language impairment. *Journal of Speech and Hearing Research, 36,* 322–337.

Davis, A.D., Sanger, D.D., & Morris-Friehe, M. (1991). Language skills of delinquent and nondelinquent adolescent males. *Journal of Communication Disorders, 24,* 251–266.

Dodge, K.A. (1985). Facets of social interaction and the assessment of social competence. In B. Schneider, K. Rubin, & J. Ledingham (Eds.), *Children's peer relations: Issues in assessment and intervention* (pp. 3–22). New York: Springer-Verlag.

Dodge, K.A., Pettit, G.S., McClaskey, C.L., & Brown, M.M. (1986). Social competence in children. *Society for Research in Child Development. Monographs, 51* (2, Serial No. 213).

Donnellan, A.M., Mirenda, P.L., Mesaros, R.A., & Fassbender, L.L. (1984). Analyzing the communicative functions of aberrant behavior. *Journal of The Association for the Severely Handicapped, 9*(3), 201–212.

Feldstein, S., & Welkowitz, J. (1978). A chronography of conversation: In defense of an objective approach. In A.W. Siegman & S. Feldstein (Eds.), *Nonverbal behavior and communication* (pp. 329–378). Hillsdale, NJ: Lawrence Erlbaum Associates.

Foster, S.L., & Ritchey, W.L. (1979). Issues in the assessment of social competence. *Journal of Applied Behavior Analysis, 12,* 625–638.

Fujiki, M., & Brinton, B. (1991). The verbal noncommunicator: A case study. *Language, Speech and Hearing Services in Schools, 22,* 322–333.

Gallagher, T.M. (1991). Language and social skills: Implications for clinical assessment and intervention with school-age children. In T.M. Gallagher (Ed.), *Pragmatics of language: Clinical practice issues* (pp. 11–41). San Diego: Singular Publishing Group.

Gallagher, T.M., & Craig, H.K. (1984). Pragmatic assessment: Analysis of a highly frequent repeated utterance. *Journal of Speech and Hearing Disorders, 49,* 368–377.

Goldstein, H., & Gallagher, T.M. (1992). Strategies for promoting the social communicative competence of young children with specific language impairment. In S.L. Odom, S.R. McConnell, & M.A. McEvoy (Eds.), *Social competence of young children with disabilities: Issues and strategies for intervention* (pp. 189–213). Baltimore: Paul H. Brookes Publishing Co.

Gottman, J.M. (1983). How children become friends. *Society for Research in Child Development. Monographs, 48*(2, Serial no. 201).

Guralnick, M.J. (1992). A hierarchical model for understanding children's peer-related social competence. In S.L. Odom, S.R. McConnell, & M.A. McEvoy (Eds.), *Social competence of young children with disabilities: Issues and strategies for intervention* (pp. 37–64). Baltimore: Paul H. Brookes Publishing Co.

Hadley, P.A., & Rice, M.L. (1991). Conversational responsiveness of speech- and language-impaired preschoolers. *Journal of Speech and Hearing Research, 34,* 1308–1317.

Hazen, N.L., & Black, B. (1989). Preschool peer communication skills: The role of social status and interaction context. *Child Development, 60,* 867–876.

Howes, C. (1990). Social status and friendship from kindergarten to third grade. *Journal of Applied Developmental Psychology, 11,* 321–330.

Hummel, L.J., & Prizant, B.M. (1993). A socioemotional perspective for understanding social difficulties of school-age children with language disorders. *Language, Speech and Hearing Services in Schools, 24,* 216–224.

Johnston, J.R. (1985). Fit, focus, and functionality: An essay on early language intervention. *Child Language Teaching and Therapy, 1*, 125–134.

Lyon, J.G. (1992). Communication use and participation in life for adults with aphasia in natural settings: The scope of the problem. *American Journal of Speech-Language Pathology: A Journal of Clinical Practice, 1*, 7–14.

MacDonald, J.D. (1989). *Becoming partners with children*. San Antonio: Special Press, Inc.

Mack, A.E., & Warr-Leeper, G.A. (1992). Language abilities in boys with chronic behavior disorders. *Language, Speech and Hearing Services in Schools, 23*, 214–223.

McTear, M.F. (1985). Pragmatic disorders: A case study of conversational disability. *British Journal of Disorders of Communication, 20*, 129–142.

Miniutti, A.M. (1991). Language deficiencies in inner-city children with learning and behavioral problems. *Language, Speech and Hearing Services in Schools, 22*, 31–38.

Odom, S.L., & McConnell, S.R. (1992). Improving social competence: An applied behavior analysis perspective. *Journal of Applied Behavior Analysis, 25*, 239–243.

Odom, S.L., McConnell, S.R., & McEvoy, M.A. (1992). Peer-related social competence and its significance for young children with disabilities. In S.L. Odom, S.R. McConnell, & M.A. McEvoy (Eds.), *Social competence of young children with disabilities: Issues and strategies for intervention* (pp. 3–35). Baltimore: Paul H. Brookes Publishing Co.

Place, K.S., & Becker, J.A. (1991). The influence of pragmatic competence on the likeability of grade-school children. *Discourse Processes, 14*, 227–241.

Prizant, B.M., Audet, L., Burke, G., Hummel, L., Maher, S., & Theadore, G. (1990). Communication disorders and emotional/behavioral disorders in children. *Journal of Speech and Hearing Disorders, 55*, 179–192.

Prizant, B.M., & Wetherby, A.M. (1990). Toward an integrated view of early language and communication development and socioemotional development. *Topics in Language Disorders, 10*, 1–16.

Prutting, C.A. (1982). Pragmatics as social competence. *Journal of Speech and Hearing Disorders, 47*, 123–134.

Reichle, J., & Johnston, S. (1993). Replacing challenging behavior: The role of communication intervention. *Topics in Language Disorders, 13*, 77–89.

Rice, M.L. (1986). Mismatched premises of the communicative competence model and language intervention. In R.L. Schiefelbusch (Ed.), *Language competence: Assessment and intervention* (pp. 261–280). San Diego: College-Hill Press.

Rice, M.L. (1993). "Don't talk to him; he's weird." A social consequences account of language and social interactions. In A.P. Kaiser & D.B. Gray (Eds.), *Communication and language intervention series: Vol. 2. Enhancing children's communication: Research foundations for intervention* (pp. 139–158). Baltimore: Paul H. Brookes Publishing Co.

Rice, M.L. (in press). Social consequences of specific language impairment. In H. Grimm & H. Skowronek (Eds.), *Language acquisition problems and reading disorders: Aspects of diagnosis and intervention*. New York: Walter DeGruyter.

Rice, M.L., Hadley, P.A., & Alexander, A.L. (in press). Social biases toward children with speech and language impairments: A correlative causal model of language limitations. *Applied Psycholinguistics*.

Rice, M.L., Sell, M.A., & Hadley, P.A. (1991). Social interactions of speech- and language-impaired children. *Journal of Speech and Hearing Research, 34*, 1299–1307.

Sameroff, A.J. (1987). The social context of development. In N. Eisenberg (Ed.), *Contemporary topics in developmental psychology* (pp. 273–291). New York: John Wiley & Sons.

Sameroff, A.J., & Chandler, M.J. (1975). Reproductive risk and the continuum of caretaking casualty. In F.D. Horowitz, M. Hetherington, S. Scarr-Salapatek, & G. Siegel (Eds.), *Review of child development research* (Vol. 4, pp. 187–244). Chicago: University of Chicago Press.

Sameroff, A., & Fiese, B. (1990). Transactional regulation and early intervention. In S. Meisels & J. Shonkoff (Eds.), *Early intervention: A handbook of theory, practice, and analysis*. New York: Cambridge University.

Semel, E., Wiig, E.H., & Secord, W. (1987). *Clinical Evaluation of Language Fundamentals–Revised: Examiner's Manual*. San Antonio: The Psychological Corporation.

Siperstein, G.N. (1992). Social competence: An important construct in mental retardation. *American Journal on Mental Retardation, 96*, iii–vi.

Snow, C. (1984). Parent–child interaction and the development of communicative ability. In R.L. Schiefelbusch & J. Pickar (Eds.), *The acquisition of communicative competence* (pp. 69–107). Baltimore: University Park Press.

Snow, C., & Ferguson, C. (Eds.). (1977). *Language acquisition and input*. Cambridge, UK: Cambridge University Press.

Tomblin, J.B., & Liljegreen, S.J. (1985). The identification of socially significant communication needs in older language-impaired children: A case example. In D.N. Ripich & F.M. Spinelli (Eds.), *School discourse problems* (pp. 219–230). San Diego: College-Hill Press.

9

Early Identification
of Reading Disabilities in Children
with Speech-Language Impairments

Hugh W. Catts, Chieh-Fang Hu,
Linda Larrivee, and Linda Swank

FOR SOME TIME RESEARCHERS AND practitioners have been interested in early identification of reading disabilities (e.g., Badian, 1982; Jansky & de Hirsch, 1972). However, progress in this area has been limited, in part, by the way we have conceptualized or defined reading disabilities. Traditional definitions of reading disabilities are exclusionary (e.g., Critchley, 1970). These definitions define the disorder by excluding factors known to be associated with learning problems in general; for example, low intelligence or sensory deficits. As such, exclusionary definitions tell us much more about what the disorder is not than what it is. The only explicitly stated symptom in most definitions is the presence of reading difficulties. Thus, when using these definitions, we must wait until a child has experienced reading problems, and frequently academic failure, before we can identify the disability. This late identification often leads to a cascade of negative consequences such as low self-concept, poor attitude toward reading, and lack of opportunities to read (Johnston & Winograd, 1985; Stanovich, 1986).

Identification of a potential reading disability need not wait until children have entered school and experienced difficulties learning to read. Developmentally, a reading disability must be more than a reading problem. There are no neurological structures or cognitive processes that are specific to reading that could fail to develop in young children (Ellis, 1985, 1987). Written language is a relatively recent development in human cultures (Rayner & Pollatsek, 1989). As a result, we have no biologic adaptations specific to reading. Rather, reading relies on cognitive (and perceptual) processes whose primary functions lie in other domains. The parasitic nature of reading has important implications for early identification of reading disabilities.

Given that reading is supported by more general cognitive abilities, we should be able to identify reading disorders on the basis of deficits in these abilities. Moreover, because reading-related cognitive abilities most likely develop early in life, it should be possible to identify potential reading problems before children enter school and are taught to read.

VISUAL FACTORS

Much research attention has been devoted to uncovering the cognitive and perceptual abilities related to reading disabilities (Kamhi & Catts, 1989; Snowling & Thomson, 1991; Stanovich, 1988; Vellutino, 1979). A common assumption is that reading disabilities are the result of visual-processing deficits. Indeed, early studies reported that poor readers often had problems with visual processing. These included difficulties in visual sequencing or orientation (Hermann, 1959; Orton, 1925), visual memory (Goyen & Lyle, 1973; Lyle & Goyen, 1968), and eye movements (Ciuffreda, Bahill, Kenyon, & Stark, 1976). Many of these early studies, however, have been criticized on the basis of serious design limitations (see Vellutino, 1979). For example, early studies often failed to control for verbal processing in visual perception or visual memory tasks. When verbal processing was controlled, apparent visual deficits in poor readers often disappeared (Vellutino, Harding, Phillips, & Steger, 1975; Vellutino, Steger, DeSetto, & Phillips, 1975) More recently, better designed investigations have been undertaken, which have uncovered other visual deficits in poor readers. These have included problems in visual persistence (DiLollo, Hanson, & McIntyre, 1983; Lovegrove, 1991; Slaghuis & Lovegrove, 1985), binocular convergence (Stein, 1989; Stein, Riddell, & Fowler, 1988), and visual crowding (Stein, 1991). Although recent work may clarify the role of visual deficits in reading disabilities, it has yet to provide strong support for specific visual factors that may be useful in early identification.

LANGUAGE BASIS

Research has also examined the language basis of reading disabilities. Unlike work on visual factors, research in this area has converged to provide strong support that language deficits underlie many reading disabilities (Kamhi & Catts, 1989; Liberman & Shankweiler, 1985; Scarborough, 1990, 1991; Vellutino, 1979). This finding should not be surprising given the role language plays in reading. Many of the cognitive processes involved in oral language comprehension are operative in reading, as well. In fact, it has often been argued that once words have been decoded or recognized, reading and listening are quite similar (e.g., Sticht & James, 1984). In accordance with this view, Gough and Tunmer (1986) have proposed a simple model of reading in which reading comprehension is considered to be the product of written word recognition and linguistic comprehension. In support of this proposal, Hoover and Gough (1990) showed that children's reading comprehension scores could be predicted quite well on the basis of their performance on tests of word recognition (reading pseudowords) and listening comprehension.

The relationship between language deficits and reading disabilities has been investigated from several perspectives. One body of research has examined language processing in children with reading disabilities. This work has shown that children with reading disabilities have problems in language processing. These problems include difficulties in the use and/or comprehension of morphology and syntax (Doehring, Trites, Patel, & Fiederowicz, 1981; Fletcher, Satz, & Scholes, 1981; Vellutino & Scanlon, 1987; Vogel, 1974), narrative production (Davenport, Yingling, Fein, Galin, & Johnstone, 1986; Feagans & Short, 1984; Roth & Spekman, 1989), and use of text-level comprehension strategies (Donahue, 1984; Short & Ryan, 1984). Language deficits of poor readers have also been observed in naming (Denckla & Rudel, 1976; Ellis, 1981; German, 1982; Kamhi, Catts, Mauer, Apel, & Gentry, 1988; Katz, 1986; Snyder & Downey, 1991; Wolf, 1986), verbal short-term memory (Brady, 1986; Cohen & Netley, 1981; Shankweiler, Liberman, Mark, Fowler, & Fisher, 1979; Torgesen & Houck, 1980), and metalinguistic awareness (Bradley & Bryant, 1983; Fox & Routh, 1983; Kamhi & Catts, 1986; Kamhi et al., 1988; Lundberg, 1982; Pratt & Brady, 1988; Vellutino & Scanlon, 1987).

Whereas the research above demonstrates a relationship between reading disabilities and language impairments, its implications for early identification are unclear. A major problem in this body of work is that language and reading abilities/disabilities were examined concurrently. That is, children were *already* demonstrating reading problems when their language abilities were investigated. As a result, it is not clear whether the observed language deficits were antecedents of reading problems (i.e., early manifestations) or consequences of reading disabilities. The latter is certainly a viable alternative. Reading is a linguistic activity and, as such, exposes children to language and language learning. Because of their reading problems, children with reading disabilities do not read as much as good readers and, thus, they have less opportunity to learn language from reading. Given this lack of opportunity, it would be predicted that children with reading disabilities would have some language problems when compared to their peers without reading disabilities (Donahue, 1986; Stanovich, 1986).

Another line of research contributing to our understanding of the language basis of reading disabilities is the longitudinal follow-up of children with preschool speech-language impairments (see Aram & Hall, 1989; Weiner, 1985 for review). Early studies in this area employed a retrospective approach in which investigators examined past clinical records and compared the results to current academic functioning (Aram & Nation, 1980; Hall & Tomblin, 1978; Strominger & Bashir, 1977). More recently, researchers have used a prospective design in which children with speech-language impairments are identified in preschool or kindergarten and subsequently tested for reading achievement in the primary grades (Bishop & Adams, 1990; Catts, 1993; Magnusson & Naucler, 1990; Menyuk, Chesnick, Liebergott, Korngold, D'Agostino, & Belanger, 1991; Stark et al., 1984; Tallal, Curtiss, & Kaplan, 1989; Wilson & Risucci, 1988). Because reading outcome in these studies was compared to speech-language problems prior to entering school, the speech-language deficits found to be related to reading disabilities might be considered to be early manifestations of or antecedents to reading disabilities. As a result, we may be able to identify children at risk for reading disabilities on the basis of the results of this research. This work is of further relevance to early identification because it involves a group of children who frequently are identified prior to beginning school. Because children with speech-language impairments often are seen during the preschool years, their risk for reading disabilities can be evaluated prior to entering school.

Follow-up studies have consistently found that children with speech-language impairments are at risk for reading disabilities (Bishop & Adams, 1990; Catts, 1993; Menyuk et al., 1991; Tallal et al., 1989). Many preschool children with speech-language impairments seem to go on to have significant problems learning to read in school. However, not all children with speech-language impairments have been found to have reading difficulties. One factor that has been shown to be related to reading outcome in these studies is the nature of the speech-language impairment. Research demonstrates that children with semantic–syntactic deficits, or what is generally referred to as a language impairment, are at a higher risk for reading disabilities than are children with problems limited to articulation or phonology (Bishop & Adams, 1990; Hall & Tomblin, 1978; Levi, Capozzi, Fabrizi, & Sechi, 1982; Shriberg & Kwiatkowski, 1988). In fact, children with articulation impairments alone may most often show normal reading development (Bishop & Adams, 1990).

Several follow-up studies have linked performance on semantic–syntactic language measures with reading achievement. Bishop and Adams (1990) identified 83 children with speech-language impairments at age 4, and tested their reading achievement in the school years. Many of these children were found to have reading problems at age 8. Bishop and Adams further reported that mean length of utterance at age $4^1/_2$ and $5^1/_2$ was a good predictor of reading ability/disability at age 8. They also found that a measure of receptive syntactic ability contributed significantly to predicting reading achievement. Similar findings have been reported by Tallal et al. (1989) in a longitudinal study of 67 children with speech-language impairments. They found that preschool measures of receptive semantic–syntactic abilities were related to reading achievement in the primary grades.

In another recent investigation, Magnusson and Naucler (1990) also found measures of semantic–syntactic language abilities to be related to reading outcome in children with speech-language impairments. The best predictors of reading achievement in these children, however, were measures of metalinguistic ability, specifically phonological awareness. Phonological awareness is the awareness that words are composed of syllables and phonemes. Magnusson and Naucler found that the ability in kindergarten to identify phonemes in words and make rhyme judgments was closely related to reading achievement in the first grade. Menyuk et al. (1991) reported similar results in a study of 130 children at risk for reading disabilities. They found standardized measures of semantic–syntactic language abilities to be significantly correlated with later reading performance. However, measures of metalinguistic abilities, including phonological awareness, were reported to be the best overall predictors of reading achievement.

Thus, the follow-up studies reviewed above indicate that measures of semantic–syntactic language abilities and measures of metalinguistic abilities may be useful in the early identification of reading disabilities. Furthermore, several studies suggest that metalinguistic measures may be the most closely related to reading outcome. However, one variable not considered in this research is how reading achievement is assessed. Various aspects of reading achievement have been measured, but attention has not been given to the relationship between different aspects of reading achievement and early language deficits. It may be that the best predictor of reading achievement in children with speech-language impairments depends upon what aspect of reading is measured.

Generally, reading achievement in young children is measured in terms of word recognition and/or comprehension abilities (Lesiak & Bradley-Johnson, 1983). Although related, word recognition and comprehension often vary within a given child (Aaron & Joshi, 1992). Some children exhibit very good word recognition but poor comprehension, whereas others have good comprehension but relatively poor decoding skills (Hoover & Gough, 1990). Thus, recognizing words and comprehending text may involve different underlying processes. As such, we might expect to find that the language measures that best predict reading achievement will depend upon whether we measure children's word recognition or their comprehension abilities.

If reading achievement is measured in terms of word recognition, language measures such as phonological awareness might be expected to be related closely to reading outcome. Phonological awareness is often argued to be a prerequisite to learning to decode words (Adams, 1990; Liberman & Shankweiler, 1985; Stanovich, 1988). Indeed, a large body of research involving children predominately without speech-language impairments has consistently shown a strong relationship between measures of word recognition and phonological awareness (Bradley & Bryant, 1985; Fox & Routh,

1983; Liberman & Shankweiler, 1985; Lundberg, Olofsson, & Wall, 1980; Stanovich, Cunningham, & Cramer, 1984; Tunmer & Nesdale, 1985; Vellutino & Scanlon, 1987; Yopp, 1988). If, however, reading is measured in terms of comprehension, language tests involving semantic–syntactic abilities should be important in predicting reading achievement. Semantic–syntactic language abilities are essential to deriving an understanding of sentences and text (Perfetti, 1985; Rayner & Pollatsek, 1989).

FOLLOW-UP INVESTIGATION

The relationship between early speech-language impairments and various measures of reading achievement was examined in a recently completed follow-up investigation (Catts, 1993). In this study, 56 children with speech-language impairments and 30 children without impairments were identified in kindergarten and tested for reading achievement in the first and second grades. In kindergarten, subjects were given a battery of speech-language measures. This battery included standardized tests of expressive and receptive semantic and syntactic abilities and a measure of articulation (see Table 1). The results of this testing indicated that 41 of the children with speech-language impairments displayed a significant language impairment. These subjects performed at least 1 standard deviation below the mean on receptive language measures and/or expressive language measures. The remaining 15

Table 1. Standardized and nonstandardized speech-language tasks administered in kindergarten

Receptive language
  Peabody Picture Vocabulary Test–R (Dunn & Dunn, 1981)
  Test of Language Development–2: Grammatical understanding
    (Newcomer & Hammill, 1988)
  Token Test for Children: Part 5 (DiSomoni, 1978)

Expressive language
  Expressive One Word Picture Vocabulary Test (Gardner, 1979)
  TOLD: Sentence imitation, grammatical closure
  Structured Photographic Expressive Language Test–2 (Weiner & Kresheck, 1983)

Articulation
  Goldman-Fristoe Test of Articulation (Goldman & Fristoe, 1986)

Phonological awareness
  Deletion
  Blending

Rapid naming
  Rapid Naming of Animals
  Rapid Naming of Objects
  Rapid Naming of Colors

subjects did not display a language impairment, according to the above criterion, but had an articulation impairment. All subjects had normal nonverbal intellectual abilities and hearing acuity.

In addition to the standardized speech-language measures, subjects were administered two measures of phonological awareness and three measures of rapid naming (see Table 1). The deletion task required subjects to repeat a word after deleting the initial syllable or phoneme. In the blending tasks, subjects blended together a series of syllables, onsets and rimes, or phonemes (cf. Catts, 1993, for examples). Finally, in the rapid-naming tasks, children were required to name rapidly a set of familiar colors, objects, or colored animals. Like phonological awareness, rapid naming has been argued to be closely linked with word recognition (Blachman, 1984; Denckla & Rudel, 1976; Wolf, 1986).

In first and second grades, subjects were given the Word Identification and Word Attack subtests of the Woodcock Reading Mastery Tests—Revised (Woodcock, 1987). These tests measured subjects' abilities to recognize words or pseudowords presented in isolation. In second grade, subjects also received the Gray Oral Reading Test–Revised (GORT–R) (Wiederholt & Bryant, 1986). This test provided a measure of speed and accuracy of word recognition in context and a measure of reading comprehension.

The results of the above study indicated that many of the subjects with speech-language impairments were having reading difficulties in first and second grades. Approximately 50% of the subjects with speech-language impairments performed 1 *SD* or more below the mean of the subjects without impairments on tests of word recognition. A similar percentage of problems was observed in reading comprehension. Whereas many subjects with speech-language impairments showed reading difficulties, others were reading at or above the mean of the subjects without impairments on tests of word recognition and comprehension.

Statistical analyses were carried out to examine factors related to variability in reading outcome in first grade. In these analyses, subjects' performances on standardized language tests were partitioned into measures of receptive semantic–syntactic language (REC LANG) and expressive semantic–syntactic language abilities (EXP LANG). REC LANG was calculated by converting subjects' performance on each of the receptive language tests to z-scores and averaging these scores. Similar procedures were employed to obtain the measure of EXP LANG. Correlational analysis showed no significant relationship between first-grade reading achievement and articulation (see Table 2). This finding was consistent with that of previous studies that have failed to find a relationship between articulation impairments and reading disabilities (Bishop & Adams, 1990; Hall & Tomblin, 1978). Group comparisons revealed further that subjects with articulation disorders alone were reading at a level similar to that of subjects without impairments. Unlike the articulation

Table 2. Pearson product–moment correlation coefficients between kindergarten measures and first-grade reading achievement

	Word ID	Word attack
REC LANG	.29[a]	NS
EXP LANG	.37	.49
Articulation	NS	NS
Deletion	.59	.60
Blending	.46	.53
Rapid Naming of Animals	.52	.42
Rapid Naming of Objects	.53	.44
Rapid Naming of Colors	.48	.35

Data presented in this table are adapted from Catts (1993).

Note: Correlation coefficients for rapid-naming tasks are expressed in absolute values rather than negative correlations.

[a]$p < .05$, all other significant correlations $p < .01$.

measure, standardized language measures were found to be related to reading in first grade. REC LANG and EXP LANG showed a low-to-moderate correlation with the Word Identification (Word ID) subtest, whereas EXP LANG had a moderate correlation with the Word Attack subtest. Higher correlations were generally found between first-grade reading achievement and phonological awareness and rapid naming.

In order to examine the relative contributions of the kindergarten measures in explaining the variance in first-grade reading achievement among the subjects with speech-language impairments, a series of hierarchical multiple regressions were performed. In these analyses, the two phonological awareness measures were combined into an overall measure of phonological awareness (PA). The three rapid-naming tasks were also combined to form a single measure of rapid naming (RAN). These measures were entered in the regression analyses with REC LANG and EXP LANG in several fixed orders (see Table 3). The results demonstrated that when the phonological awareness and rapid-naming measures were entered before the other language measures, they accounted for a large amount of variance in first-grade reading achievement. Once PA and RAN were entered into the regression analyses, REC LANG and EXP LANG accounted for no significant amount of variance in Word ID and only a small amount of variance in Word Attack. When entered before PA and RAN, the EXP LANG and REC LANG did account for a significant amount of variance in first-grade reading measures. However, a large amount of variance remained and was explained in part by the phonological awareness and rapid-naming measures. Thus, the phonological awareness and rapid-naming measures were better predictors of first-grade tests of word recognition than were measures of receptive and expressive language ability.

Similar analyses were carried out on the reading achievement data from second grade. Table 4 shows that phonological awareness and rapid-naming measures were again moderately correlated with reading achievement. As was generally the finding in first grade, the semantic–syntactic language measures

Table 3. R^2 change in fixed order multiple regression analyses for first-grade reading achievement

Steps in regression	Reading achievement	
	Word ID	Word attack
1. PA	.32	.37
2. RAN	.12	.05[a]
3. REC LANG	NS	NS
4. EXP LANG	NS	.05[a]
1. REC LANG	.10[a]	NS
2. EXP LANG	NS	.24
3. RAN	.18	.10
4. PA	.12	.13

Data presented in this table are adapted from Catts (1993).

Note: Nonverbal IQ was entered in regression analyses prior to the language measures.

[a]$p < .05$, all other R^2 changes $p < .01$.

were related less to Word ID and Word Attack than were the phonological awareness and rapid-naming measures. However, the semantic–syntactic language measures showed comparable correlations to phonological awareness and rapid naming in the case of the GORT–R speed and accuracy measure and higher correlations in the case of the GORT–R comprehension measure.

Hierarchical multiple regression analyses were also performed on second-grade reading achievement (see Table 5). The results of these analyses were similar to those in first grade for the measures of word recognition (i.e., Word ID, Word Attack, and GORT–R Speed/Accuracy). In the regression analyses involving word recognition, phonological awareness and rapid-naming tasks were better predictors than were measures of receptive and expressive language. Once PA and RAN were entered in the regression analyses for word recognition, REC LANG and EXP LANG did not account for a significant amount of variance. The results were quite different for reading

Table 4. Pearson product–moment correlation coefficients between kindergarten measures and second-grade reading achievement

	Word ID	Word attack	GORT–R (S/A)	GORT–R (C)
REC LANG	.31[a]	.37	.52	.71
EXP LANG	.42	.46	.59	.69
ARTIC	NS	NS	NS	NS
Deletion	.55	.63	.61	.56
Blending	.39	.55	.45	.50
RANAN	.51	.46	.45	.35[a]
RANOBJ	.54	.56	.63	.46
RANCOL	.48	.43	.53	.40

Data presented in this table are adapted from Catts (1993).

Note: GORT–R (S/A) = Speed and accuracy score from the Gray Oral Reading Tests–Revised. GORT–R (C) = Comprehension score from the Gray Oral Reading Test–Revised. Correlation coefficients for rapid-naming tasks expressed in absolute values rather than negative correlations.

[a]$p < .05$, all other significant correlations $p < .01$.

Table 5. R^2 changes in fixed order multiple regression analyses for second-grade reading achievement

	Reading achievement			
Steps in regression	Word ID	Word attack	GORT–R (S/A)[a]	GORT–R (C)
1. PA	.23	.36	.26	.25
2. RAN	.14	.10	.16	.07[a]
3. EXP LANG	NS	NS	NS	.09
4. REC LANG	NS	NS	NS	.06[a]
1. EXP LANG	.15	.17	.26	.33
2. REC LANG	NS	NS	NS	.07
3. RAN	.16	.14	.14	.04[a]
4. PA	.07[a]	.16	.04[a]	NS

Data presented in this table are adapted from Catts (1993).

Note: Nonverbal IQ was entered in regression analyses prior to the language measures. GORT–R (S/A) = Speed and accuracy score from the Gray Oral Reading Test–Revised. GORT–R (C) = Comprehension score from the Gray Oral Reading Test–Revised.

[a]$p < .05$, all other significant R^2 changes $p < .01$.

comprehension. In this case, the measures of receptive and expressive language were better predictors than were the phonologic awareness and rapid-naming measures. REC LANG and EXP LANG explained a large amount of independent variance in reading comprehension. PA and RAN, however, accounted for less variance in reading comprehension than they did in word recognition. However, RAN continued to provide a small, but independent, contribution to predicting reading comprehension.

IMPLICATIONS FOR EARLY IDENTIFICATION

The results of the longitudinal study detailed above are consistent with those of previous investigations (Bishop & Adams, 1990; Menyuk et al., 1991; Tallal et al., 1989). Our work, as well as that of others, demonstrates a strong relationship between early speech-language impairments and reading disabilities. Many children with speech-language impairments during preschool or kindergarten have been shown to have reading problems in the early school years. This research suggests, therefore, that speech-language impairments may be the early manifestations of a reading disability. In other words, these impairments may precede and foretell a subsequent reading disability. As such, early speech-language impairments may be used to identify potential reading problems prior to children entering school and subsequently having difficulty learning to read.

The research reviewed above further suggests that certain speech-language impairments are more closely related to reading problems than others. Specifically, deficits in semantic–syntactic aspects of language are more often associated with subsequent reading disabilities than are articulation or phonological problems. In fact, our work, as well as that of others (e.g.,

Bishop & Adams, 1990), indicates that children with articulation problems alone may be at no more risk for reading disabilities than are children without a history of speech-language impairments. Apparently, the ability to produce the sounds of language accurately is not a necessary skill for learning to read.

Unlike children with articulation impairments, children with language impairments are at high risk for reading problems. Consistent with this finding is the observation that measures of semantic and syntactic abilities are good predictors of reading achievement in children with speech-language impairments. Studies also show that measures of phonological awareness and rapid naming are related to reading achievement. Thus, these various language measures may be useful in the early identification of reading disabilities in children with speech-language impairments. Our research demonstrates, however, that the specific relationship between these measures of early language ability and reading achievement will depend upon how reading achievement is measured.

In the early school grades, reading achievement is often assessed by tests of word recognition. Our work indicates that when reading achievement is measured in terms of word recognition, the best predictors of reading outcome will be measures of phonological awareness and rapid naming. Children with speech-language impairments who have good phonological awareness and good rapid-naming skills in kindergarten will perform well on measures of word recognition in the early school grades. However, children with poor phonological awareness and poor rapid naming will more likely have problems learning to decode and recognize words.

The findings above are consistent with a large body of research predominately involving children without speech-language impairment. Research has shown that preschool measures of phonological awareness and rapid naming are closely linked with early word recognition skills (Blachman, 1984; Bradley & Bryant, 1985; Stanovich, 1988; Wolf, 1984). These findings have led to the position that deficits in phonological awareness and rapid naming lie near the core of the reading problems manifested in the early school grades (Catts, 1989a, 1989b; Stanovich, 1988; Wagner & Torgesen, 1987). As a result, measures of phonological awareness and rapid naming may prove to be effective predictors of reading outcome in a wide range of children, not just children with speech-language impairment.

Reading achievement is also often assessed in terms of reading comprehension. Our research indicates that when reading achievement is assessed in this manner, children's semantic–syntactic language abilities become important in predicting reading outcome. Young children with good semantic–syntactic language abilities should do well subsequently in reading comprehension, whereas, those with poor language abilities will likely have problems in reading comprehension. Our results indicate that these predictions for reading comprehension may hold true as early as the second grade.

Measures of rapid naming and phonological awareness may also contribute independently to predicting reading comprehension, especially in the early school grades. In the initial stages of learning to read, not only will semantic and syntactic language skills influence the understanding of a text, but word recognition abilities will also have a significant effect on reading comprehension. (Gough & Tunmer, 1986). Young children with poor word recognition skills, for example, may not recognize enough words to comprehend adequately what they read. Thus, because of their relationship to word recognition, rapid-naming and phonological awareness skills should contribute independently to predicting reading comprehension in the early school grades. Our results, however, showed that such independent contribution was limited to a rather modest effect, involving only rapid naming. It was unclear why phonological awareness did not also contribute independently to explaining variance in reading comprehension. Therefore, future investigators must consider further the role of such factors as phonological awareness and rapid naming in predicting reading comprehension in the early school grades.

In conclusion, follow-up studies of children with speech-language impairments have begun to identify early language deficits that are predictive of subsequent reading disabilities. Standardized language measures currently available may be used to identify some of these deficits. In the case of other deficits, nonstandardized testing instruments must be employed. Future investigations must move toward the standardization of these measures and their validation in predicting reading disabilities in young children.

REFERENCES

Aaron, P.G., & Joshi, R.M. (1992). *Reading problems: Consultation and remediation.* New York: Guilford Press.

Adams, M.J. (1990). *Beginning to read: Thinking and learning about print.* Cambridge, MA: MIT Press.

Aram, D., & Hall, N. (1989). Longitudinal follow-up of children with preschool communication disorders: Treatment implications. *School Psychology Review, 18,* 487–501.

Aram, D., & Nation, J. (1980). Preschool language disorders and subsequent language and academic difficulties. *Journal of Communication Disorders, 13,* 159–179.

Badian, N. (1982). The prediction of good and poor readers before kindergarten entry: A four-year follow-up. *Journal of Special Education, 16,* 309–318.

Blachman, B. (1984). Relationship of rapid-naming ability and language analysis skill to kindergarten and first-grade reading achievement. *Journal of Educational Psychology, 76,* 610–622.

Bishop, D., & Adams, C. (1990). A prospective study of the relationship between specific language impairment, phonological disorders, and reading retardation. *Journal of Child Psychology & Psychiatry, 31,* 1027–1050.

Brady, S. (1986). Short-term memory, phonological processing, and reading ability. *Annals of Dyslexia, 36,* 138–153.

Bradley, L., & Bryant, P. (1983). Categorizing sounds and learning to read: A casual connection. *Nature, 30,* 419–421.

Bradley, L., & Bryant, P. (1985). *Rhyme and reason in reading and spelling.* International Academy for Research in Learning Disabilities Monograph Series, No. 1. Ann Arbor: University of Michigan Press.

Catts, H.W. (1989a). Phonological processing deficits and reading disabilities. In A. Kamhi, & H. Catts (Eds.), *Reading disabilities: A developmental language perspective.* Newton, MA: Allyn & Bacon.

Catts, H.W. (1989b). Defining dyslexia as a developmental language disorder. *Annals of Dyslexia, 39,* 50–64.

Catts, H.W. (1993). The relationship between speech-language impairments and reading disabilities. *Journal of Speech and Hearing Research, 36,* 948–958.

Ciuffreda, K.J., Bahill, A.T., Kenyon, R.V., & Stark, L. (1976). Eye movements during reading: Case studies. *American Journal of Optometry and Physiological Optics, 53,* 389–395.

Cohen, R., & Netley, C. (1981). Short-term memory deficits in reading disabled children, in absence of opportunity for rehearsal strategies. *Intelligence, 5,* 69–76.

Critchley, M. (1970). *The dyslexic child.* Springfield, IL: Charles C Thomas.

Davenport, L., Yingling, C.D., Fein, G., Galin, D., & Johnstone, J. (1986). Narrative speech deficits in dyslexics. *Journal of Clinical and Experimental Neuropsychology, 8,* 347–361.

Denckla, M., & Rudel, R. (1976). Rapid automatized naming (R.A.N.): Dyslexia differentiated from other learning disabilities. *Neuropsychologia, 14,* 471–479.

DiLollo, V., Hanson, D., & McIntyre, J.S. (1983). Initial stages of visual information processing in dyslexia. *Journal of Experimental Psychology: Human Perception and Performance, 9,* 923–935.

DiSomoni, F. (1978). *The Token Test for Children.* Boston: Teaching Resource Corporation.

Doehring, D.G., Trites, R.L., Patel, P.G., & Fiederowicz, C.A.M. (1981). *Reading disabilities: The interaction of reading, language, and neuropsychological deficits.* New York: Academic Press.

Donahue, M. (1984). Learning disabled children's conversational competence: An attempt to activate the inactive listener. *Applied Psycholinguistics, 5,* 21–35.

Donahue, M. (1986). Linguistic and communicative development in learning-disabled children. In S. Ceci (Ed.), *Handbook of cognitive, social, and neuropsychological aspects of learning disabilities* (pp. 263–289). Hillsdale, NJ: Lawrence Erlbaum.

Dunn, L.M., & Dunn, L.M. (1981). *Peabody Picture Vocabulary Test–Revised.* Circle Pines, MN: American Guidance Service, Inc.

Ellis, A.W. (1985). The cognitive neuropsychology of developmental (and acquired) dyslexia: A critical survey. *Cognitive Neuropsychology, 2,* 169–205.

Ellis, A.W. (1987). Review: On problems in developing cognitively transmitted cognitive modules. *Mind & Language, 2,* 242–251.

Ellis, N.C. (1981). Visual and name coding in dyslexic children. *Psychological Research, 43,* 201–218.

Feagans, L., & Short, E. (1984). Developmental differences in the comprehension and production of narratives by reading-disabled and normally achieving children. *Child Development, 55,* 1727–1736.

Fletcher, J.M., Satz, P., & Scholes, R. (1981). Developmental changes in the linguistic performance correlates of reading achievement. *Brain and Language, 13,* 78–90.

Fox, B., & Routh, D. (1983). Reading disability, phonemic analysis, and dysphonetic spelling: A follow-up study. *Journal of Clinical Child Psychology, 12,* 28–32.

Gardner, M.F. (1979). *Expressive One Word Picture Vocabulary Test.* Novato, CA: Academic Therapy Publications.

German, D. (1982). Word-finding substitutions in children with learning disabilities. *Language, Speech and Hearing Services in Schools, 13,* 223–230.

Goldman, R., & Fristoe, M. (1986). *Goldman-Fristoe Test of Articulation.* Circle Pines, MN: American Guidance Service, Inc.

Gough, P., & Tunmer, W. (1986). Decoding, reading, and reading disability. *Remedial and Special Education, 7,* 6–10.

Goyen, J.D., & Lyle, J. (1973). Short-term memory and visual discrimination in retarded readers. *Perceptual and Motor Skills, 36,* 403–408.

Hall, P., & Tomblin, J. (1978). A follow-up study of children with articulation and language disorders. *Journal of Speech and Hearing Disorders, 43,* 227–241.

Hermann, K. (1959). *Reading disability.* Copenhagen: Munksgaard.

Hoover, W., & Gough, P. (1990). The simple view of reading. *Reading and Writing: An Interdisciplinary Journal, 2,* 127–160.

Jansky, J., & de Hirsch, K. (1972). *Preventing reading failure: Prediction, diagnosis, intervention.* New York: Harper & Row.

Johnston, P.H., & Winograd, P.N. (1985). Passive failure in reading. *Journal of Reading Behavior, 17,* 279–301.

Kamhi, A.G., & Catts, H.W. (1986). Toward an understanding of developmental language and reading disorders. *Journal of Speech and Hearing Disorders, 51,* 337–347.

Kamhi, A.G., & Catts, H.W. (1989). *Reading disabilities: A developmental language perspective.* Newton, MA: Allyn & Bacon.

Kamhi, A.G., Catts, H.W., Mauer, D., Apel, K., & Gentry, B. (1988). Phonological and spatial processing abilities in language- and reading-impaired children. *Journal of Speech and Hearing Disorders, 53,* 316–327.

Katz, R. (1986). Phonological deficiencies in children with reading disability: Evidence from an object-naming task. *Cognition, 22,* 225–257.

Lesiak, J., & Bradley-Johnson, S. (1983). *Reading assessment for placement and programming.* Springfield, IL: Charles C Thomas.

Levi, G., Capozzi, F., Fabrizi, A., & Sechi, E. (1982). Language disorders and prognosis for reading disabilities in developmental age. *Perceptual and Motor Skills, 54,* 1119–1122.

Liberman, I., & Shankweiler, D. (1985). Phonology and the problems of learning to read and write. *Remedial and Special Education, 6,* 8–17.

Lovegrove, W. (1991). Spatial frequency processing in normal and dyslexic readers. In J. Stein (Ed.), *Visual dyslexia: Vol. 13. Vision and visual dysfunction* (pp. 148–154). London: Macmillan.

Lundberg, I. (1982). Linguistic awareness as related to dyslexia. In Y. Zotterman (Ed.), *Dyslexia: Neuronal, cognitive, and linguistic aspects.* Wenner-Gren Symposium, Vol. 35.

Lundberg, I., Olofsson, A., & Wall, S. (1980). Reading and spelling skills in the first school years predicted from phonemic awareness skills in kindergarten. *Scandinavian Journal of Psychology, 21,* 159–173.

Lyle, J.G., & Goyen, J. (1968). Visual recognition, developmental lag, and strephosymbolia in reading retardation. *Journal of Abnormal Psychology, 73,* 25–29.

Magnusson, E., & Naucler, K. (1990). Reading and spelling in language-disordered children—linguistic and metalinguistic prerequisites: Report on a longitudinal study. *Clinical Linguistics and Phonetics, 4,* 49–61.

Menyuk, P., Chesnick, M., Liebergott, J., Korngold, B., D'Agostino, R., & Belanger, A. (1991). Predicting reading problems in at-risk children. *Journal of Speech and Hearing Research, 34,* 893–903.

Newcomer, P.L., & Hammill, D.D. (1988). *Test of Language Development–2 Primary.* Austin, TX: PRO-ED.

Orton, S.T. (1925). "Word-blindness" in school children. *Archives of Neurology, 14,* 581–615.

Perfetti, C. (1985). *Reading ability.* New York: Oxford University Press.

Pratt, A.E., & Brady, S. (1988). Relation of phonological awareness to reading disability in children and adults. *Journal of Educational Psychology, 80,* 319–323.

Rayner, K., & Pollatsek, A. (1989). *The psychology of reading.* Englewood Cliffs, NJ: Prentice Hall.

Roth, F.P., & Spekman, N.J. (1989). Higher-order language processes and reading disabilities. In A.G. Kamhi & H.W. Catts (Eds.), *Reading disabilities: A developmental language perspective* (pp. 159–197). Newton, MA: Allyn & Bacon.

Scarborough, H. (1990). Very early language deficits in dyslexic children. *Child Development, 61,* 1728–1743.

Scarborough, H. (1991). Early syntactic development of dyslexic children. *Annals of Dyslexia, 41,* 207–220.

Shankweiler, D., Liberman, I.Y., Mark, L.S., Fowler, C.A., & Fisher, F.W. (1979). The speech code and learning to read. *Journal of Experimental Psychology: Human Learning and Memory, 5,* 531–545.

Short, E., & Ryan, E. (1984). Metacognitive differences between skilled and less skilled readers: Remediating deficits through story grammar and attribution training. *Journal of Educational Psychology, 76,* 225–235.

Shriberg, L., & Kwiatkowski, J. (1988). A follow-up study of children with phonologic disorders of unknown origin. *Journal of Speech and Hearing Disorders, 53,* 144–156.

Slaghuis, W.L., & Lovegrove, W.J. (1985). Spatial-frequency-dependent visible persistence and specific reading disability. *Brain and Cognition, 4,* 219–240.

Snowling, M., & Thomson, M. (1991). *Dyslexia: Integrating theory and practice.* London: Whurr Publishers, Ltd.

Snyder, L.S., & Downey, D.M. (1991). The language-reading relationship in normal and reading-disabled children. *Journal of Speech and Hearing Research, 34,* 129–140.

Stanovich, K. (1986). Matthew effects in reading: Some consequences of individual differences in the acquisition of literacy. *Reading Research Quarterly, 19,* 278–303.

Stanovich, K. (1988). The right and the wrong places to look for the cognitive locus of reading disability. *Annals of Dyslexia, 38,* 154–180.

Stanovich, K., Cunningham, A., & Cramer, B. (1984). Assessing phonological awareness in kindergarten children: Issues of task comparability. *Journal of Experimental Child Psychology, 38,* 175–190.

Stark, R., Bernstein, L., Condino, R., Bender, M., Tallal, P., & Catts, H. (1984). Four-year follow-up study of language-impaired children. *Annals of Dyslexia, 34,* 49–68.

Stein, J.F. (1989). Unstable vergence control and specific reading impairment. *British Journal of Ophthalmology, 73,* 49.

Stein, J.F. (1991). Vision and language. In M. Snowling & M. Thomson (Eds.), *Dyslexia: Integrating theory and practice.* London: Whurr Publishers, Ltd.

Stein, J.F., Riddell, P., & Fowler, M.S. (1988). Disordered vergence eye movement control in dyslexic children. *British Journal of Ophthalmology, 72,* 162–166.

Sticht, T.G., & James, J.H. (1984). Listening and reading. In D. Pearson (Ed.), *Handbook of reading research* (Vol. 1, pp. 293–317), New York: Longman.

Strominger, A.Z., & Bashir, A. (1977). *A nine-year follow up of language-delayed children.* Paper presented at the annual convention of the American Speech-Language-Hearing Association, Chicago.

Tallal, P., Curtiss, S., & Kaplan, R. (1989). *The San Diego longitudinal study: Evaluating the outcomes of preschool impairment in language development.* Final Report, National Institute of Neurological Communication Disorders.

Torgeson, J., & Houck, D. (1980). Processing deficiencies of learning-disabled children who perform poorly on the digit span test. *Journal of Educational Psychology, 72,* 141–160.

Tunmer, W., & Nesdale, A. (1985). Phonemic segmentation skill and beginning reading. *Journal of Educational Psychology, 77,* 417–427.

Vellutino, F.R. (1979). *Dyslexia: Theory and research.* Cambridge, MA: MIT Press.

Vellutino, F.R., Harding, C.J., Phillips, F., & Steger, J.A. (1975). Differential transfer in poor and normal readers. *Journal of Genetic Psychology, 126,* 3–18.

Vellutino, F., & Scanlon, D. (1987). Phonological coding, phonological awareness, and reading ability: Evidence from a longitudinal and experimental study. *Merrill-Palmer Quarterly, 33,* 321–363.

Vellutino, F.R., Steger, J.A., DeSetto, L., & Phillips, F. (1975). Immediate and delayed recognition of visual stimuli in poor and normal readers. *Journal of Experimental Child Psychology, 19,* 223–232.

Vogel, S.A. (1974). Syntactic abilities in normal and dyslexic children. *Journal of Learning Disabilities, 7,* 103–109.

Wagner, R., & Torgesen, J. (1987). The nature of phonological processing and its causal role in the acquisition of reading skills. *Psychological Bulletin, 101,* 192–212.

Weiner, E.O., & Kresheck, J.D. (1983). *Structured Photographic Expressive Language Test-2.* Sandwich, IL: Janelle Publications, Inc.

Weiner, P.S. (1985). The value of follow-up studies. *Topics in Language Disorders, 5,* 78–92.

Wiederholt, J.C., & Bryant, B.R. (1986). *Gray Oral Reading Test-Revised.* Austin, TX: PRO-ED.

Wilson, B., & Risucci, D. (1988). The early identification of developmental language disorders and the prediction of the acquisition of reading skills. In R. Masland & M. Masland (Eds.), *Preschool prevention of reading failure* (pp. 187–203). Parkton, MD: York Press.

Wolf, M. (1984). Naming, reading, and the dyslexias: A longitudinal overview. *Annals of Dyslexia, 34,* 87–136.

Wolf, M. (1986). Rapid alternating stimulus naming in the developmental dyslexias. *Brain and Language, 27,* 360–379.

Woodcock, R.W. (1987). *Woodcock Reading Mastery Tests–Revised.* Circle Pines, MN: American Guidance Service, Inc.

Yopp, H. (1988). The validity and reliability of phoneme awareness tests. *Reading Research Quarterly, 23,* 159–177.

10

Reconsideration of IQ
Criteria in the Definition
of Specific Language Impairment

Marc E. Fey, Steven H. Long, and Patricia L. Cleave

Aʟᴛʜᴏᴜɢʜ sᴘᴇᴄɪꜰɪᴄ ʟᴀɴɢᴜᴀɢᴇ ɪᴍᴘᴀɪʀᴍᴇɴᴛ ʜᴀs been the subject of much investigative scrutiny since the 1970s, the disorder is still defined largely in exclusionary terms. Children with specific language impairment (SLI) have significant delays in the development of semantic, syntactic, phonological, and/or pragmatic abilities in the relative absence of frank neurological damage, emotional disorder, or hearing loss. Another criterion that is part of virtually every definition of specific language impairment is performance IQ of no more than 1 standard deviation below the mean (i.e., performance IQs of 85 or above). When the intellectual abilities of children with SLI are evaluated, it is critical that the task be as independent of language performance as possible. Optimally, this would involve cognitive tasks that do not require verbal instructions, internalized verbal mediation, or a verbal response. Such tasks are difficult to conceive and to carry out, however (see Johnston, 1992; Johnston & Ellis Weismer, 1983). Minimally, tasks should require limited or no verbal instructions and a nonverbal response. The use of *IQ* or *intelligence* in this chapter refers to performance intelligence as determined by measures of cognition that meet these minimal requirements (e.g., Kamhi, Minor, & Mauer, 1990).

The motivation for excluding children with known neurological disturbances, severe emotional disorders, or hearing loss is relatively clear. These

This research was sponsored in part by the Ministry of Community and Social Services, Ontario. This funding was administered by the Research and Program Evaluation Unit in cooperation with the Ontario Mental Health Foundation and was funded from the MCSS Research Grants Program. We also gratefully acknowledge equipment contributions from the Ontario District Association of the Society for the Preservation of Barbershop Quartet Singing in America (the Barbershoppers). Able research assistance was provided by Kit Dench, Lynn Dupuis, Sarah Hawkins, David Loyst, Dan MacDougald, Chris Matthews, Cathy Moran, Sheila Murray, Anna Ravida, Brenda Ushiki, and Joanne Wickware.

factors may be directly responsible for the children's language-learning disorders and are likely to have a direct effect on the manner in which the affected children learn language. Where organic or readily identifiable emotional factors are involved, however, it is difficult to distinguish between those parts of the language-learning problem that are due directly to the known etiological factors and those due to other unknown factors. Therefore, exclusion of children with neurological, emotional, or hearing disorders from the group of children with specific language impairments seems justified (cf. Aram, 1992).

Rationales for including normal intelligence as a criterion for specific language impairment are much less clear. Our concerns apply to all children with intellectual deficits at least as low as the range of mild mental retardation (i.e., IQs = 55–69) who do not have frank neurological, emotional, or sensory impairments and who exhibit language performance lower than predicted by their performance mental age. In principle, the arguments presented in this chapter may be extended to *all* children with a significant mental age (MA)-language performance discrepancy but without neurological, emotional, or sensory disorders, even children with IQs below 55. Within this population, specific language impairment could be viewed as that part of a child's linguistic deficit not accounted for by the child's measured cognitive limitations.

There is evidence, however, that the causes of mental retardation are the same as those that lead to variability of intelligence in the normal IQ range. In contrast, the factors that cause severe mental retardation seem to differ from those found within the normal range (Broman, Nichols, Shaughnessy, & Kennedy, 1987; Tomblin, 1991). Therefore, we might reasonably expect the incidence of such accepted exclusionary variables as organic deficiencies to be more common in the population of individuals with IQs below 55. In this chapter, however, we restrict our arguments to that group of children with IQs of 70–85, sometimes referred to as the *borderline range* of intelligence.

It is possible to criticize the use of IQ as a criterion for specific language impairment on numerous psychometric and theoretical grounds. For example, standard error of measurement virtually is never taken into consideration when IQ criteria are applied. A child with a score of 85 who qualifies as SLI may have a "true score" of only 80. Similarly, a child who scores 78 on one day may have a true score on that test of 85. In both of these cases, the children would be categorized inappropriately. These and other criticisms are reviewed by Lahey (1990) and extended by Cole, Dale, and Mills (1992). The arguments put forward in this chapter hold even under ideal circumstances in which intelligence-test users could be completely confident of the reliability and validity of test scores.

There are at least four reasons for excluding these children with borderline intelligence in definitions of specific language impairment. First, children with lower IQs may have less specific language problems than those of children with average-performance intelligence. For example, although some children in the borderline range of intelligence have significant discrepancies between language performance and performance IQ, they may be more likely to have other problems, such as attentional or perceptual deficits, that are related directly to their language-learning problems. Stark and Tallal (1981) cited this as a factor in their SLI exclusionary criterion of performance IQ of at least 85.

It may be true that children with below-average IQs are more likely than children with average IQs to have additional cognitive deficits associated with their language impairments. But considerable evidence suggests that children with SLI are not specifically impaired in the sense that their learning problems are exclusive to language (Johnston, 1988, 1992, chap. 7, this volume; Leonard, 1987). For example, Tallal and her colleagues (Tallal, 1990; Tallal, Stark, Kallman, & Mellits, 1981; Tallal, Stark, & Mellits, 1985) have argued that children with specific language impairment display deficits in rapid temporal analysis and processing that are not restricted to language or even to the auditory modality. Deficits also have been reported in areas of cognitive development such as symbolic play (Rescorla & Goossens, 1992; Roth & Clark, 1987; Terrell, Schwartz, Prelock, & Messick, 1984) and mental imagery (Johnston & Ellis Weismer, 1983; Kamhi, 1981). While acknowledging that poor performance on representational and symbolic tasks may be partially a reflection of poor linguistic abilities, Johnston (1992) argues that children with specific language impairment display cognitive deficits in nonverbal functioning as well. The gap between the nonlinguistic cognitive abilities of children with SLI and their linguistic performance is interesting and important. Moreover, it begs for explanation, but it seems clear that children with conventionally defined SLI have problems that cut across many areas of cognitive functioning. Therefore, children with SLI cannot be distinguished clearly from children with SLI in the borderline IQ range solely on the grounds that their language learning difficulties are "pure."

The second reason for an exclusionary criterion of IQ in a definition of specific language impairment is to limit intersubject variability in research investigations. Intelligence is known to be related to the developing language performance of children. By setting the lower boundary for IQ at 85, investigators can reduce the variability in language performance that may be associated with large differences in IQ. Although this is a sensible and valuable research strategy, it is important to note that any criterion set for this research purpose is purely arbitrary. There is no conceptual or theoretical basis for selecting 85 over some other criterion, such as 70, 80, or 100. Furthermore, in practice, the setting of some arbitrary *lower* boundary for IQ will have only a limited effect on reducing variance, unless it is accompanied by an upper boundary. In fact, most definitions of specific language impairment for research purposes are biased in the manner with which they limit variation in intelligence. For example, in their survey of the literature, Camarata and Swisher (1990) found that in 49% of studies of children with SLI, IQ criteria consisted only of a report of a negative history of retardation or a lower boundary cutoff score (e.g., an IQ of 85). Even in studies in which means and standard deviations for IQ are provided, it is unusual to find an a priori upper boundary criterion for IQ. Thus, the emphasis is more on excluding children with below-average intelligence than on reducing overall variance due to variation in performance intelligence.

This emphasis creates some problems, however. It seems possible, if not likely, that a child with SLI and an IQ of 90 would have as much or more in common with a child with language impairment whose IQ is 75 (i.e., a difference of 1 standard deviation) than with another child with language impairment whose IQ is 120 (i.e., a difference of 2 standard deviations). However, whereas the child with an IQ of 120 would be considered SLI, the child with an IQ of 75 would not be. This makes sense only if it can be shown that the child with language impairment with a below-average IQ has a language profile or a language-learning style different from the child with the above-average intelligence. To date, no such demonstration has appeared. Therefore, although this practice is virtually never employed, it is possible to limit variance due to cognitive factors in research by using both upper and lower IQ limits. Even if this were done, however, the boundaries for SLI would still be arbitrary, and they would have no theoretical or conceptual basis.

A third reason for excluding children with IQs below 85 from the category of children with SLI is that these children may be fundamentally different from children with traditionally defined SLI in their linguistic profiles and/or their language-learning capabilities. For example, Kamhi and Johnston (1982) demonstrated that language delays of children with mental retardation are qualitatively different from delays of children with classically defined SLI, matched by mental age. Still, there have been numerous reports of children with mental retardation who exhibit language abilities that are lower than predicted based on their nonlinguistic cognitive skills (e.g., Fowler, Gelman, & Gleitman, 1980, cited in Kamhi & Johnston, 1982; Miller, 1988; Miller, Chapman, & MacKenzie, 1981). These deficits may require the same types of explanations needed to understand specific language impairments in children with normal intelligence. Indeed, if language-learning abilities can be impaired to a greater extent than other areas of performance, it is difficult to conceive how or why children with borderline intelligence could be immune to such impairments. Although the study of specific language impairment may require identification of subjects whose linguistic development is not complicated by intellectual and associated deficits, it seems that a definition of specific language impairment must leave open the possibility that the condition exists in children functioning at different levels of the IQ continuum.

The fourth reason for excluding children on the basis of IQ is that, if children with below-normal IQs really differ fundamentally from children with classically defined SLI, they may respond differently to intervention. Different types of intervention may be required for these children than for children with SLI who have normal IQs.

In our view, the third and fourth justifications for excluding children with below-average IQs from the population of children with SLI are the best reasons for doing so, at least when the purpose is to define the essential characteristics of the population. Children who meet all the criteria for specific language impairment but who have below normal IQs may, indeed, have linguistic profiles that differ from those of children with average intelligence scores. If they do, it may well be that these children need different types of intervention programs than those that benefit children with SLI who have average performance intelligence. These are empirical issues of the type that must be addressed if we are to develop a coherent definition of SLI that emphasizes inclusionary, rather than exclusionary, criteria. These are precisely the issues that we have begun to examine within the context of a broader study of the effectiveness of early language intervention.

Our research was designed primarily to evaluate two closely related approaches to the facilitation of grammar among children with language impairment. One program was administered by a speech-language pathologist. The other was implemented by the child's parent, who was trained in the use of intervention procedures by the speech-language pathologist. These programs were designed to employ many features that have been hypothesized or demonstrated to be effective in fostering the acquisition and/or use of individual linguistic forms over relatively short time intervals. Our investigation served to evaluate constellations of these procedures operating together over a longer period of time.

Our research interests primarily have been in children whose language-learning problems are not confounded by frank neurological symptoms, physical anomalies, emotional disorders, or mental retardation. In designing our study, however, we were well aware of the difficulties encountered in amassing a large group of subjects with SLI, especially for participation in a longitudinal investigation. Therefore, we decided from the outset to extend our criterion for performance IQ below 85. Specifically, we decided to include children with IQ scores on the Leiter International Performance Scale (Leiter, 1979) as low as 70, or 2 standard deviations below the mean. We saw no clear reason why children who met all the criteria for SLI but were functioning in the borderline range of intelligence should be expected to differ from a group of children with traditionally defined SLI in their response to our intervention. Therefore, we hypothesized that there would be no differences in the language profiles of these two groups of children or in their responses to the interventions we planned to test. We made no effort to treat IQ as a factor in our experiment, and we assigned our subjects to experimental groups at random. Still, our intervention study has given us a post hoc opportunity to begin to test our hypotheses.

We describe the subjects who participated in the larger intervention study and summarize briefly the results of the first 5-month phase of our intervention approaches (Fey, Cleave, Long, & Hughes, 1993). This provides a perspective for our examination of issues related to the IQ criterion for identifying children with SLI. After presenting the major results of the principal study, we compare subsets of subjects from the major investigation to address two additional questions. First, did subjects with IQs within the average IQ range differ from subjects in the borderline range of intelligence in their linguistic profiles prior to the investigation? Second, did the subjects from these groups differ in their responses to intervention?

STUDY 1

The subjects in the principal investigation were 30 children between the ages of 3;8 and 5;10 (see Fey et al., 1993, for specific details on subjects and group assignment). Initially, six children were assigned randomly to the *clinician intervention* group, and five children were chosen randomly to receive the *parent intervention*. These subjects were first to receive the 4½-month intervention. An additional nine children were assigned at random to a *delayed intervention* group. After a 5-month waiting period, four of the children in the *delayed intervention* group received intervention from the *clinician*. Four other *delayed intervention* subjects received the *parent intervention*. These eight children made up the second subgroups to receive the interventions. The parents of the ninth child in the *delayed intervention* group withdrew their child from the study after the waiting period because of unanticipated scheduling conflicts. After the completion of intervention for the *delayed intervention* subjects, 10 additional subjects were identified for a third intervention trial. Five of these subjects were assigned at random to *clinician intervention* and five were assigned to *parent intervention*.

For the purposes of the major experimental questions, the first and third subgroups, who received intervention immediately after identification, were combined to form the *clinician* and *parent* subgroups (ns = 11 and 10, respectively). The *delayed intervention* subjects (n = 9) served as controls.

Subject Description

The results of the pre-experimental battery for each experimental group are summarized in Table 1. On the basis of clinical observation and standardized test performance, each subject was judged to have a clinically significant impairment of expressive grammar by at least two ASHA-certified speech-

Table 1. Pre-experimental statistics for each experimental group

Intervention groups		Age (mos)	TACL–R[a] (Z)	PPVT–R[b] (Standard)	IQ[c] (Standard)	DSS[d]	PD[e]
Clinician	M	54.72	−0.35	93.73	97.09	4.22	34.00
	SD	6.05	1.11	12.26	19.55	1.36	13.08
Parent	M	56.20	−0.66	89.90	100.00	4.38	32.60
	SD	7.21	1.19	15.15	14.17	1.44	18.56
Delayed	M	55.90	−1.02	86.70	96.10	4.66	37.56
	SD	5.95	1.10	18.73	18.04	1.45	15.37

[a] Test for Auditory Comprehension of Language–Revised (Carrow-Woolfolk, 1985).
[b] Peabody Picture Vocabulary Test–Revised (Dunn & Dunn, 1981).
[c] Based on the Leiter International Performance Scale (Leiter, 1979).
[d] Developmental sentence scores (Lee, 1974) for 30-minute pre-experimental sample.
[e] Phonological Deviancy Score from the Assessment of Phonological Processes–Revised (Hodson, 1986).

language pathologists. Each child was identified minimally by a Developmental Sentence Score (DSS, Lee, 1974) below the 10th percentile for the lower of chronological or mental age. Thus, regardless of whether the child's performance IQ fell between the range of 70–84 or above 85, a discrepancy between performance in expressive grammar and performance intelligence was obtained for all subjects.

Based on their interactions with their parents and one of the examiners, all the subjects exhibited social-conversational profiles of "active conversationalists" (Fey, 1986). Our impressions of these children as appropriately assertive and responsive were further verified by parental report of the children's interactions with peers at home and at school. Although some children were clearly more assertive and responsive than others, it was determined that none required intervention programs in which the primary focus was to facilitate conversational assertiveness or responsiveness.

There were no statistically significant differences between the groups on any pre-experimental measure. This includes parent and family variables such as parent age, years of education, number of siblings, and birth order.

Intervention Programs

All intervention sessions were conducted by a master's-level speech-language pathologist (PLC) with 2 years post-master's clinical experience, who was certified by all relevant American and Canadian professional organizations. Details regarding the frequency and duration of intervention sessions for each intervention group are given in Table 2.

The parent program was designed to take less clinician time than the clinician program. Its implementation took only approximately 53% of the time required to administer the clinician intervention program.

It should be noted that no effort was made to equate the amount of intervention received by the children in the two intervention groups. Within

Table 2. Clinician time involvement for the clinician and parent interventions

	Clinician intervention	Parent intervention
Group sessions	2 hours/week (20 weeks)	2 hours/week (first 12 weeks) 2 hours/month (last 8 weeks)
Individual sessions (time per child)	1 hour/week (20 weeks)	1 hour/month (first 12 weeks) 1/2 hour/month (last 8 weeks)

the parent group, there was no reliable way to control the amount of intervention received by each child. All parents were encouraged first to use the intervention procedures at specific times and then to use them throughout the day, whenever relevant opportunities arose. Our primary concern was to evaluate the effects of these two intervention *packages* as they actually might be administered clinically. It was not our intention at any point to determine whether parents or clinicians are more effective in administering language intervention programs.

A detailed description of the parent and clinician intervention approaches is beyond the scope of this report (see Fey et al., 1993), but a brief summary is in order. For both programs, a cyclical goal-attack strategy was used. Each child began with a set of four individually selected specific goals. These goals were presented in a cyclical fashion with one goal targeted each week. When the child began to use a target productively in the group sessions for the clinician intervention group or in the monthly clinic sampling sessions for the parent intervention group, that goal either was dropped from the program or combined with other existing related goals.

Both programs relied primarily on the use of focused stimulation procedures (see Fey, 1986; Fey et al., 1993). This involved following a child's attentional lead and providing high concentrations of pragmatically appropriate models of the child's weekly target form. Wherever possible, child sentences were recast in various ways to highlight target forms.

There was one major difference between the two approaches other than the intensity of intervention and the intervention agent. Each individual clinician intervention session began with a highly structured activity that involved imitation of the target for the week as well as of a language form that was contrastive with the target. This imitation activity was designed to draw the child's attention to the target form. This usually consumed about 10 minutes of the individual session. No prompts for imitation were presented at any other time in either of the intervention approaches. This interventionist-oriented activity was not paralleled in any manner in the parent intervention program.

It should be clear that the two programs involved combining a number of procedures and strategies into packages that we believed from the outset would be effective. We were particularly interested in testing the viability of intervention approaches that made extensive use of focused stimulation procedures and a cyclical goal-attack strategy. However, our experimental design was not structured to enable us to discern the unique contribution of any individual part of the intervention packages.

Effectiveness of the Interventions

The first experimental question concerned the effectiveness of the interventions; specifically, "Were the parent- or clinician-administered interventions more effective than no intervention over a 4½-month time period?" The second question was concerned with the existence of differences in the effects of the two intervention packages.

All dependent measures used for assessing intervention efficacy were based on 30-minute interactions between the child and one of his or her primary caregivers. In all cases, the same parent or guardian interacted with the child pre- and post-experimentally.

The DSS, a general measure of grammatical development, was selected as the primary dependent variable. Increases in DSS scores arise from more frequent production of acceptable grammatical forms in any of eight categories and/or accurate production of forms in these categories, which typically are produced by developmentally older children. To help specify the nature of any observed intervention effects, three of the eight categories were selected as secondary measures. These were mean main verb score per sentence (i.e., total main verb score/number of sentences scored), mean personal pronoun score per sentence (i.e., total personal pronoun score/number of sentences scored), and percentage of sentences awarded a sentence point.

The major findings from this investigation can be summarized as follows. First, both parent and clinician intervention groups made significant gains in expressive grammar relative to the delayed intervention controls as indexed by overall DSS, mean main verb score/sentence, and percentage of sentences receiving a sentence point. Thus, the intervention had a significant effect on the children's grammatical performance. In particular, the effect for main verbs indicates that the children who received intervention either produced more complex verb forms, produced appropriate verb forms more frequently, or both as a result of the intervention. The gains in sentence points suggest that both interventions resulted in the children's production of higher proportions of sentences that were semantically and grammatically well formed.

The second major finding of this study was that there were no significant differences between the two intervention groups on any of the four DSS measures employed. Finally, more detailed analyses of the performance of individual subjects and intervention subgroups revealed that the gains made by the clinician intervention group were consistent across intervention trials. For example, the mean gains for each of the three clinician intervention subgroups clustered around the total group mean gain of 1.25 DSS points. In contrast to this balanced performance across intervention trials, the distribution of gains for the parent intervention subjects was bimodal—subjects tended to make either very large gains or very limited gains on the DSS variables. Thus, although the parent intervention was shown to have a powerful overall group effect, there was greater variability and less consistency in gains for subjects who received this intervention than for subjects who received the clinician intervention. The reasons for these differences across parent intervention subgroups were not apparent from our study of pre-experimental and intervention variables (see Fey et al., 1993, for further details).

STUDY 2

The first question of concern for our post hoc investigation was whether subjects in Study 1 with IQs in the borderline range of intelligence (BI subjects) differed in their linguistic profiles from subjects with average intelligence (AI subjects) prior to intervention. Of the 30 subjects included in the study, 8 had Leiter IQs between 70 and 84. To make valid and meaningful comparisons, it was important to have subject groups that were similar on cognitive and gross linguistic parameters. Therefore, the ranges of mental ages (MAs) and mean lengths of utterance (MLUs) found in the group of eight BI subjects were determined. The MAs of these subjects ranged from 36 to 54 months, and the MLUs ranged between 1.86 and 4.25. Ten AI subjects had both MAs and MLUs within these ranges, and all ten were included in the subsequent analyses.

These two groups of children were compared on a number of linguistic and nonlinguistic variables, using t tests for independent groups. As shown in Figure 1, the BI subjects tended to be older, although this difference was not quite statistically significant, $t(1,16) = 1.77$, $p = .096$. As planned, their performance IQs were markedly lower than those of the AI subjects, $t(1,16) = 5.61$, $p = .00004$. Despite the restriction placed on the range of MAs in the AI group, however, the mean MA for the BI subjects was still significantly lower than that for the AI subjects, $t = 2.07 (1,16)$, $p = .055$. The difference in raw scores for the PPVT–R was not statistically significant ($p = .184$), but the advantage of the AI group for the TACL–R approached significance, $t = 1.92 (1,16)$, $p = .073$. As planned, the groups were roughly equivalent for MLU. Although the groups were equivalent for MLU, the BI children tended to be older and lower in MA and in auditory

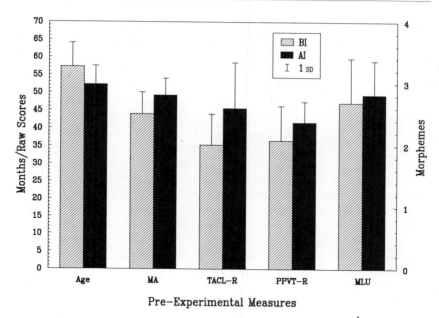

Figure 1.   Pre-experimental characteristics of subjects in the borderline (BI) and average (AI) intelligence groups.

comprehension as measured by TACL–R. Thus, the gap between MA and language performance seemed to be not as great for the BI subjects as for the AI subjects.

We compared these groups of children on all measures employed in Study 1: DSS, mean main verb score/sentence, mean personal pronoun score/sentence, and average sentence points awarded. The differences between groups were nonsignificant on all measures ($ps > .39$). However, Johnston and Kamhi (1984) found that a signature component of the performance of children with SLI was a high frequency of errors. Therefore, we examined the possibility that one of the groups made more errors than the other. The results of these analyses showed that, although the percentage of errors for main verbs was high for both groups, the error rates across groups did not differ significantly ($M = 45.8\%$ for BI and 40.2% for AI, $p = .38$). In general, the pronoun errors were much less frequent for both groups and there were no differences between groups in pronoun error frequency ($M = 15.3\%$ for BI and 17% for AI, $p = .79$).

Our analyses of expressive grammar do not represent an exhaustive examination of the grammatical systems of these two groups of children. Still, the areas that were evaluated and the measures used were those that have distinguished children with traditionally defined SLI from other children with language-learning problems (Johnston & Kamhi, 1984; Leonard, 1972; Liles

& Watt, 1984). The present analyses show that the AI and BI subjects came from the same population of children with language impairment.

Despite the similarities between the subjects at the outset of the experiment, however, it is still possible that there were differences in the ways in which the children responded to intervention. For example, it is possible that the mild level of intellectual impairment that resulted in borderline Leiter scores would interfere with the BI children's ability to profit from a package of procedures designed and tested primarily on children who were functioning typically and children with classically defined SLI. Leonard (1983) recognized the potential of using observed differences in children's response to intervention as the basis for subclassifying children with language-learning problems. Therefore, the next step in the investigation was to compare AI and BI subjects at the end of the 4½-month intervention program.

One of the BI subjects did not take part in intervention because of scheduling problems. Therefore, the groups to be tested initially consisted of 10 AI subjects and 7 BI subjects. Some children in each group had served as delayed intervention subjects in the principal investigation. To examine the effects of intervention, the pre-experimental scores for these children were their scores *following* the 5-month control period at the testing point immediately *before* intervention. The postintervention scores were the scores at the testing point immediately *after* the 4½-month intervention period. Thus, for all children, tests of the effects of intervention involve scores before and after the 4½-month period during which they received intervention.

The two groups were compared on DSS and percentage Sentence Points awarded. In addition, three measures of main verb performance were employed— mean main verb score per sentence, percentage error in the main verb category, and average complexity of verbs produced correctly. The third main verb measure involves calculating the total number of points in the DSS main verb category and dividing this number by the number of items that received a score. Thus, inappropriate attempts at target structures do not figure into this measure.

The gains made by both groups across the 5-month period were statistically significant for all these measures, as determined by t-tests for related samples ($ts > 2.06$, $ps < .07$). Univariate analyses of covariance were then performed to compare the performances of the AI and BI groups. In each case, the same variable measured immediately prior to intervention served as the covariate. None of the small differences observed between groups was statistically significant, however ($ps > .5$). This finding suggests that the BI subjects responded to the intervention in the same positive manner as did the AI subjects.

It is important to recall that subjects who received the parent intervention and those who received the clinician intervention were collapsed into the AI and BI groups for these analyses. We know from the results of the larger study, however, that there was more consistency in the effects of the clinician intervention. If the AI and BI subjects were not distributed equally across the two intervention groups, this could have had an important effect on our results.

In fact, six of the AI subjects received the parent intervention, whereas only two of the BI children received parent intervention. Therefore, it seemed prudent to determine whether the finding of no differences between the AI and BI groups following intervention would hold up if we examined only the clinician intervention subjects. For these comparisons, there were five BI subjects and four AI subjects. These two groups were equivalent in MLU. As was the case in previous comparisons, however, the BI children tended to have lower MAs than the AI subjects (Mann-Whitney U test = 3.0, $Z = -1.71, p = .086$). Thus, the expressive grammar/MA gaps were not quite as great for the BI subjects as they were for the AI subjects.

These two groups were then compared on their responses to the 4½-month clinician intervention. The results of a Mann-Whitney U test revealed that the DSS gains of the BI group ($M = 1.44$) were, in fact, significantly greater than those of the AI group ($M = 1.11$), U = 0, $Z = -2.45, p = .014$. This effect is illustrated in Figure 2. Both groups made marked gains, but the improvements of the BI subjects were especially large and highly consistent across the five subjects. Examination of the children's gains on main-verb measures and percentage of sentence points awarded provided no clear-cut clues as to the nature of the differences in DSS gains. As shown in Figure 3,

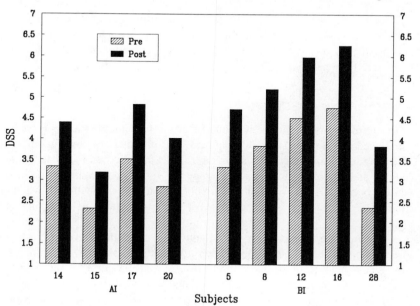

Figure 2.   Pre- and postintervention DSSs for AI and BI subjects.

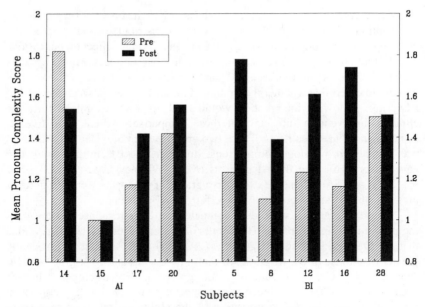

Figure 3. Mean pre- and postintervention pronoun complexity scores for AI and BI subjects.

however, the BI children made greater gains in the average complexity of the pronouns they used.

Given the large number of tests that were run, these findings of group differences may be purely spurious. It is not inconceivable, however, that because the BI children had less significant delays relative to their MAs, they were able to benefit more from the type of intervention they received.

SUMMARY AND CONCLUSIONS

In the primary investigation, we found that the two intervention approaches were effective in facilitating development of expressive grammar in children with language impairment. This finding reveals that focused stimulation procedures and a cyclical goal-attack strategy are viable components of an intervention package. However, our data do not permit a determination of whether each of these features was necessary, or even important, in rendering the observed effects.

Furthermore, the primary investigation showed that the effects of the intervention were more consistent when it was administered by the clinician. This result should *not* be interpreted to mean that the clinician intervention was inherently better than that of the parents. In fact, the children who made the greatest gains in the entire experiment came from the parent intervention group. Rather, the result suggests that the intervention was administered more consistently, and probably more deftly, across children by the clinician working directly with the children than it was by the parents. This is not too surprising, perhaps. But in light of this finding, it is especially clear that clinicians who undertake parent training programs must find ways to evaluate carefully the effects of their intervention, just as they are urged to do with direct forms of intervention. When the children are not responding positively, clinicians must be prepared to modify the program in some ways. Among these should be consideration of some direct clinician contact with the child.

Our comparisons of children with language impairment and IQs in the normal and borderline ranges suggest that, despite measurable differences in performance intelligence, when they are matched roughly by MA and MLU, these children have similar grammatical systems and respond to grammatical intervention in ways that are essentially the same.

There are a number of limitations to our post hoc study, several of which must be considered when evaluating our results and conclusions. First, attempts were made to render the groups equivalent in both MA and MLU by restricting the MA and MLU range for the AI subjects. Although this method yielded groups that were equivalent for MLU, the BI subjects were still lower in MA. This indicates that their language impairments, when referenced to MA, were somewhat less severe than those of the AI subjects. Had the groups been equated for MA as well as MLU, there might have been differences in the DSS profiles of the subjects who were not observed in this investigation. Second, the primary linguistic difference observed in these studies was that the BI subjects who received clinician intervention made greater DSS gains than did the AI subjects who received the same intervention. This difference may be entirely spurious, or it may be due to the smaller discrepancy between MA and expressive syntax for the BI subjects or to some other factor. Third, only one measure of intelligence was used to evaluate the children's intellectual abilities. It is possible that other standardized tests or nonstandardized procedures would have led to different classifications of the children and, therefore, different results. Finally, DSS variables were used almost exclusively in our analyses of these children's grammatical abilities. DSS measures have been used to uncover qualitative differences in the expressive language of typically developing children and children with SLI (Johnston & Kamhi, 1984; Leonard, 1972; Liles & Watt, 1984). Therefore, their use in this study seemed well founded. However, many additional aspects of grammatical and semantic ability might have been included. It is possible that differences between groups might have been revealed had other measures been used.

To address these methodological weaknesses, studies should be planned to compare the language profiles and the language-learning abilities of children with conventionally defined SLI, older children with language impairment and varying degrees of below-normal intelligence who have significant MA–language discrepancies, and younger typically developing children. The subjects should be matched by general measures of linguistic and nonlinguistic cognitive abilities. They should then be compared on a number of grammatical, semantic, phonological, and pragmatic measures and in their response to various types of intervention.

Based on our investigation and on our experience with children whose language skills are lower than could be predicted by their borderline IQ scores, we suspect that such studies will reveal no differences, at least between the AI and BI subjects. We further suspect that as long as a significant MA–language performance gap exists in the absence of frank neurological, emotional, or sensory impairments, children at various levels of intelligence will exhibit profiles of extremely limited grammatical morphology (e.g., limited use of auxiliaries and verb inflections, see Leonard, 1989) and in morphology learning that distinguish them from younger, typical language learners. This is because we believe that these children with language impairment come from the same population of impoverished language learners.

This speculation should not be taken as an argument that IQ and other nonlinguistic exclusionary criteria are inappropriate or irrelevant in studies of children with SLI. Minimizing variance and reducing potential confounds in our studies and clearly describing subject profiles will always be important aspects of investigations of children with SLI. But we believe that the arbitrary criterion of performance IQ of 85 or greater, which is employed as a method of research, has lulled many of us into thinking that this standard has special relevance in defining this population of children. The results of our preliminary studies suggest that this is a mistake that may lead us to focus our attention on exclusionary criteria as identifying attributes instead of intensifying our efforts to discover the linguistic and nonlinguistic features that set this group of poor language learners apart from all others.

REFERENCES

Aram, D.M. (1992). Brain injury and language impairment in childhood. In P. Fletcher & D. Hall (Eds.), *Specific speech and language disorders in children: Correlates, characteristics and outcomes* (pp. 80–93). San Diego: Singular Publishing Group.

Broman, S., Nichols, P.L., Shaughnessy, P., & Kennedy, W. (1987). *Retardation in young children: A developmental cognitive.* Hillsdale, NJ: Lawrence Erlbaum.

Camarata, S., & Swisher, L. (1990). A note on intelligence assessment within studies of specific language impairment. *Journal of Speech and Hearing Research, 33,* 205–207.

Carrow-Woolfolk, E. (1985). *Test for Auditory Comprehension of Language.* Allen, TX: DLM Teaching Resources.

Cole, K., Dale, P., & Mills, P. (1992). Stability of the intelligence quotient–language quotient relation: Is discrepancy modeling based on a myth? *American Journal of Mental Retardation, 97,* 131–143.

Dunn, L.M., & Dunn, L.M. (1981). *The Peabody Picture Vocabulary Test–Revised.* Circle Pines, MN: American Guidance Service.

Fey, M.E. (1986). *Language intervention with young children.* San Diego: College-Hill Press.

Fey, M.E., Cleave, P.L., Long, S.H., & Hughes, D.L. (1993). Two approaches to the facilitation of grammar in language-impaired children: An experimental evaluation. *Journal of Speech and Hearing Research, 36,* 141–157.

Fowler, A., Gelman, R., & Gleitman, L. (1980, October). *A comparison of normal and retardate language equated with MLU.* Paper presented at the 5th Annual Children's Language Conference, Boston.

Hodson, B. (1986). *The Assessment of Phonological Processes–Revised.* Danford, IL: Interstate Press.

Johnston, J.R. (1988). Specific language disorders in the child. In N. Lass, L. McReynolds, J. Northern, & D.E. Yoder (Eds.), *Handbook of speech-language pathology and audiology* (pp. 685–715). Toronto, Ontario, Canada: B.C. Decker.

Johnston, J.R. (1992). Cognitive abilities of language-impaired children. In P. Fletcher, & D. Hall (Eds.), *Specific speech and language disorders in children: Correlates, characteristics, and outcomes* (pp. 105–116). San Diego: Singular Publishing Group.

Johnston, J.R., & Ellis Weismer, S. (1983). Mental rotation abilities in language-disordered children. *Journal of Speech and Hearing Research, 26,* 397–403.

Johnston, J.R., & Kamhi, A.G. (1984). The same can be less: Syntactic and semantic aspects of the utterances of language-impaired children. *Merrill-Palmer Quarterly, 30,* 65–86.

Kamhi, A.G. (1981). Nonlinguistic symbolic and conceptual abilities of language-impaired and normally developing children. *Journal of Speech and Hearing Research, 24,* 446–453.

Kamhi, A.G., & Johnston, J.R. (1982). Towards an understanding of retarded children's linguistic deficiencies. *Journal of Speech and Hearing Research, 25,* 435–445.

Kamhi, A.G., Minor, J.S., & Mauer, D. (1990). Content analysis and intratest performance profiles on the Columbia and the TONI. *Journal of Speech and Hearing Research, 33,* 375–379.

Lahey, M. (1990). Who shall be called language disordered? Some reflections and one perspective. *Journal of Speech and Hearing Disorders, 55,* 612–620.

Lee, L. (1974). *Developmental sentence analysis.* Evanston, IL: Northwestern University Press.

Leiter, R. (1979). *Leiter International Performance Scale.* Chicago: Stoelting Company.

Leonard, L.B. (1972). What is deviant language? *Journal of Speech and Hearing Disorders, 37,* 315–340.

Leonard, L.B. (1983). Discussion: Part II: Defining the boundaries of language disorders in children. In J.F. Miller, D. E. Yoder, & R.L. Schiefelbusch (Eds.), *Contemporary issues in language intervention* (pp. 107–112). Rockville, MD: The American Speech-Language-Hearing Association.

Leonard, L.B. (1987). Is specific language impairment a useful construct? In S. Rosenberg (Ed.), *Advances in applied psycholinguistics: Vol. 1. Disorders of first-language development* (pp. 1–39). New York: Cambridge University Press.

Leonard, L.B. (1989). Language learnability and specific language impairment in children. *Applied Psycholinguistics, 10,* 179–202.

Liles, B., & Watt, J. (1984). On the meaning of "language delay." *Folia Phoniatrica, 36,* 40–48.

Miller, J.F. (1988). The developmental asynchrony of language development in children with Down syndrome. In L. Nadel (Ed.), *The psychobiology of Down syndrome* (pp. 168–198). Cambridge, MA: MIT Press.

Miller, J.F., Chapman, R., & MacKenzie, H. (1981). Individual differences in the language acquisition of mentally retarded children. *Proceedings from the Second Wisconsin Symposium on Research in Child Language Disorders, 2,* 130–146.

Rescorla, L., & Goossens' M. (1992). Symbolic play development in toddlers with expressive specific language impairment. *Journal of Speech and Hearing Research, 35,* 1290–1302.

Roth, F.P., & Clark, D.M. (1987). Symbolic play and social participation abilities of language-impaired and normally developing children. *Journal of Speech and Hearing Disorders, 52,* 17–25.

Stark, R.E., & Tallal, P. (1981). Selection of children with specific language deficits. *Journal of Speech and Language Disorders, 46,* 114–122.

Tallal, P. (1990). Fine-grained discrimination deficits in language-learning impaired children are specific neither to the auditory modality nor to speech perception. *Journal of Speech and Hearing Research, 33,* 616–617.

Tallal, P., Stark, R.E., Kallman, C., & Mellits, D. (1981). A reexamination of some nonverbal perceptual abilities of language-impaired and normal children as a function of age and sensory modality. *Journal of Speech and Hearing Research, 24,* 351–357.

Tallal, P., Stark, R.E., & Mellits, D. (1985). Identification of language-impaired children on the basis of rapid perception and production skills. *Brain and Language, 25,* 314–322.

Terrell, B. Y., Schwartz, R.G., Prelock, P.A., & Messick, C.K. (1984). Symbolic play in normal and language-impaired children. *Journal of Speech and Hearing Research, 27,* 424–429.

Tomblin, J.B. (1991). Examining the cause of specific language impairment. *Language, Speech and Hearing Services in Schools, 22,* 69–74.

Author Index

Subject Index

Page numbers followed by "t" or "f" indicate tables or figures, respectively.